Herbal Pharmacology in the People's Republic of China

A Trip Report of the American Herbal Pharmacology Delegation

Submitted to the
Committee on Scholarly Communication
with the People's Republic of China

NATIONAL ACADEMY OF SCIENCES
Washington, D.C. 1975

NOTICE

The project that is the subject of this report was approved by the Governing Board of the National Research Council, whose members are drawn from the Councils of the National Academy of Sciences, the National Academy of Engineering, and the Institute of Medicine. The members of the Committee responsible for the report were chosen for their special competence and with regard for appropriate balance.

This report has been reviewed by a group other than the authors according to procedures approved by a Report Review Committee consisting of members of the National Academy of Sciences, the National Academy of Engineering, and the Institute of Medicine.

Library of Congress Catalog Card No. 75-39772
International Standard Book No. 0-309-02438-2

Available from:
Printing and Publishing Office
National Academy of Sciences
2101 Constitution Avenue, N.W.
Washington, D.C. 20418

Printed in the United States of America

TABLE OF CONTENTS

PREFACE

The Committee on Scholarly Communication with the People's Republic of China sponsored the visit of a twelve-member Herbal Pharmacology Study Group to the People's Republic of China from June 1 to June 26, 1974. In China, the group was hosted by the Chinese Medical Association. This report is a compilation of the findings of the group members, whose task was to discuss research on natural products for therapeutic use, identification of medically effective elements, and development of synthetic drugs with those elements. The group visited Peking, Tientsin, Shanghai, Nanking, Hangchow, and Kwangchow.

The Committee on Scholarly Communication with the People's Republic of China is sponsored jointly by the American Council of Learned Societies, the National Academy of Sciences, and the Social Science Research Council. It was formed in 1966 to promote scholarly communication between the two countries in the natural sciences, medical sciences, social sciences, and humanities.

INTRODUCTION

During the month of June 1974, twelve U.S. specialists in chemistry, medicine, pharmacology, pharmacognosy, pharmacy, and Chinese culture visited a series of major Chinese cities for the purpose of assessing the current status of herbal pharmacology (both basic and clinical) in the People's Republic of China.* We hoped, by visiting medical schools (both traditional+ and Western-type), research institutes, hospitals, pharmacies, pharmaceutical plants, and plantations, to learn something about current Chinese approaches to the use of herbal medicines and to the detailed study of such medicines in man and animals, as well as to identify types of plant materials that might justify prompt attention from Western scientists and physicians interested in developing important new drugs from natural products.

Our group was selected with the following points in mind: (1) a complement of scientific disciplines appropriate to our mission; (2) geographic distribution so as to include scholars from different areas, schools, and institutes in the United States; (3) representation of academia, industry, and government; and (4) the presence in the delegation of China scholars as well as scientists with a working knowledge of the Chinese language. Scholars who had visited the People's Republic of China in the previous 5 years were not considered.

Problems

It soon became obvious that certain factors - some predictable and others not - were to make our mission more difficult than many of us had suspected. One of the first of these was inseparability of politics and medicine in China. No society possesses a scientific establishment independent of non-scientific forces in the culture, but the relationships in China seem especially complex.

---

*The itinerary and the Chinese whom we met are listed in the Appendix.

+By "traditional medicine" we mean the mixture of traditional Chinese medical practices with Western training methods that is now called "Chinese medicine" (Chung-i) in the People's Republic of China.

In the People's Republic politics takes command, and science is made to serve the people. Great emphasis is placed upon the need for technological self-reliance, and scientists are taught that they must combine what is useful from the West with native devices and discoveries in order to meet the needs of the nation. In pharmacological work this effort is expressed in Mao Tse-tung's formula calling for the union of Western and Chinese medicine.

Pharmacology particularly lends itself to this attempted union because of classical China's rich materia medica and pharmacopoeia. The Chinese consistently refer to their herbal remedies as being "the product of two thousand years of the people's struggle against disease," and cite the millennial endurance of these medicines as adequate empirical proof of their effectiveness. Yet Chinese drug therapy did not emerge from an empirical tradition based on pharmacological properties alone. Magic and ritual also played a large role in drug formulas, and abstract cosmological terms distinguished the Chinese traditional cures from simple folk medicine. As historians of Chinese science have remarked:

> The heterogeneous character of Chinese materia medica begins to make sense only when we realize that the tradition of the great pharmacopoeias (which is parallel to that of the great theoretical and therapeutic treatises) is anything but folk medicine. It is a comprehensive and highly rational body of theory and practice held together by the most fundamental concepts of classical natural philosophy, which have been refined, modified, and elaborated to incorporate the phenomena of health and sickness.[1]

The very fact that the materia medica was so closely linked with Confucian cosmogony gravely jeopardized traditional medical practitioners when China began a selective process of modernization in the late nineteenth century. As more and more Western-style physicians were trained in the twentieth century, and as Confucianism itself came to be seen as an expression of China's "backward" and "feudal" *ancien régime*, traditional Chinese medicine was attacked for being superstitious and nonscientific. Although traditional doctors continued to abound, their status remained outside the regular medical profession during the years of Kuomintang (Nationalist) rule. In areas controlled by the Chinese Communist Party, however, traditional physicians were mildly encouraged by the authorities, and Chinese herbal medicines were manufactured to supplement modern pharmaceuticals.

The Chinese Communists initially supported traditional medicine because Chinese-style physicians were an important available resource and because the tradition itself seemed to stem from popular folk roots. At that time, the Party's leadership intended to westernize traditional practitioners - not sinify Western-style doctors. In 1944 Chairman Mao urged modern doctors to "unite with and help reform Chinese doctors,"[2] and five years later, when the People's Republic was established, Chinese-style physicians were encouraged to elevate the standards of their own profession. Western-style doctors nonetheless continued to dominate clinical and laboratory research. Although the Minister of Culture in 1950 urged that the two styles of medicine be united, the traditionalists were denied research centers as well as membership in the Chinese Medical Association.

In 1954, however, there was a dramatic shift in emphasis. After launching a campaign to exalt traditional medicine, the government founded research institutes to explore this valuable cultural legacy, and in 1956 it implemented a policy to train more Chinese-style physicians. These moves were opposed by some Western-style physicians. In 1957 the Dean of Pharmacy at Peking Medical College accused the Ministry of Public Health of "dragging pharmaceutics back to the eighteenth century,"[3] and there were many other signs that traditional physicians remained second-class professionals in the eyes of modernists. Yet the government continued to support traditional medicine and, during the Great Leap Forward in 1958, initiated programs to train Western-style doctors in Chinese medicine. These programs continued through the Cultural Revolution (1966-1970) and were strengthened under the aegis of the campaign to criticize Confucius and Lin Piao (the former Minister of Defence who plotted against Mao Tse-tung). As we shall see later in this report, the marriage of Western and Chinese medicine still shows signs of strain, though divorce certainly seems unlikely in the near future.

One major cause of continued strain is the theoretical incompatibility of Western and purely traditional medical systems. As Cooper and Sivin have pointed out:

> Modern medicine evolved in the closest possible consonance with a scientific method that originated in physics. Chinese medicine is a rational construction originated from basic conceptions of the universe and its microcosm, man. Data taken from experience were systematically worked into a metaphysical structure that could be neither buttressed nor destroyed by experimental proof.[4]

Because of a fundamentally different approach, it is extremely difficult for Western-trained scientists (whether native Chinese or foreign visitors) to evaluate the products of a medical tradition that lacked the idea of experimental control and a metaphysical system that defied empiric rejection.

> Traditional Chinese medicine strove to treat the whole person rather than his isolated parts, and to think of him in relation to his emotional sphere and physical environment. This ancient diagnostic and therapeutic approach in many respects anticipates that of the sophisticated modern doctor. But the criteria that the Chinese physician used to verify effectiveness of a treatment were drastically different from those of modern scientific medicine - although perhaps less easily distinguishable from the attitudes and rules of thumb current

> in the broad areas of medical application in which doctors are still willing to credit anything that seems to work regardless of the demands of systematic verification. More to the point in attempting to understand Chinese practice are its criteria of disproof, which appear to have been particularly permissive.[5]

But this does not mean that herbal remedies cannot be pharmacologically tested, nor that the Chinese themselves are unconcerned with verifying their efficacy. Contemporary Chinese-style physicians are given Western training, and their research institutes employ modern techniques to analyze drugs. However, their experiments are devoted more to the validation of the efficacy of traditional medicines than to the isolation of their active principles. And that, too, forms part of what might be called a Maoist strategy of drug development. Such a strategy owes a great deal to Mao Tse-tung's theory of practice.

> Knowledge starts with practice, reaches the theoretical planes via practice, and then has to return to practice. The active function of knowledge not only manifests itself in the active leap from perceptual knowledge to rational knowledge, but also - and this is the more important - in the leap from rational knowledge to revolutionary practice.... This is the process of testing and developing theory, the continuation of the whole process of knowledge.[6]

Practice confirms theoretical knowledge, which in turn is regarded as useful only if it proves itself in practice. Although the importance of theory is by no means denied, Maoism is inclined to value the social usefulness of technical knowledge and to deprecate pure theory or basic science as such. Distrustful of mere experts, Maoists constantly urge the scientist to put his knowledge to the test of practice; and in the field of pharmacology this often means leaping over laboratory study of the physiologic basis for drug action to move directly into clinical testing. This means, from a utilitarian point of view, that if a drug appears to have beneficial effects, valuable time and resources need not be devoted to elaborate chemical experiments isolating its active principles.

Chinese clinical evaluation does not involve the kinds of controlled experiments often used in the West - and this, too, is partly a reflection of political concerns. In revolutionary Chinese medicine nothing is ideally more sacred than the welfare of the patients, who are supposed to be kept totally informed about the medical measures being taken to cure them. It is thus politically and professionally immoral for a physician to do anything other than provide the best possible medical treatment with the full knowledge of the patient. Double-blind experiments are ruled out, and placebos may not be administered. (A similar objection to the use of placebos has recently surfaced in Western countries, such as France.) This policy conforms to socialist ideals, but it does not entirely satisfy foreign pharmacologists, who - while relatively culture-free - still possess a bias toward values characteristic of the West since the Scientific Revolution.

Nevertheless, Western scientists who have been privileged to visit China recognize the pragmatic reasons behind this seemingly hit-or-miss search for clinically effective drugs in the traditional materia medica. Inspired by the Maoist doctrine of self-reliance, Chinese medical workers and scientists both manufacture their own versions of Western pharmaceuticals whenever possible and conduct major programs to find new and inexpensive drugs in the traditional materia medica without excessive investment in laboratory research.

Among the problems our delegation faced in China was also that of language. The time consumed in translation, the obstacle it provided to spontaneous and free-flowing discussion (for most of the members of the delegation), and the accuracy of the translation were all sources of concern to us. Occasionally, a lengthy and heated discussion among our Chinese colleagues was distilled and presented to us in a surprisingly brief manner, making us wonder what had been lost in the translation. Fortunately, the Chinese-speaking members of the delegation could often set us right about the precise meaning of the Chinese terms that had been used in the discussions.

A related problem was the misunderstandings arising out of the use of different words to describe the same thing or the same word to describe different things. The semantic problems we encountered were substantial. It took quite a while to realize that words like "antipyretic" and "cardiotonic" were not what they seemed. In discussion with foreigners, the Chinese use these words as verbal shorthand, which, like our scientific jargon, is not always an aid to communication. "Febrifuge" and "antipyretic" to us characterize measures that lower abnormally high body temperature. Not so to the Chinese, for whom the terms refer to remedies that decrease body "heat" in the ancient sense of a "humor" or "essence" or "principle" present in superfluity but not necessarily measured by a thermometer. "Diuretic" (when applied to traditional drugs) means "to decrease humidity." "Cardiotonic" was in a sense more confusing - at times it was used as we would use it, to denote an improvement in cardiac contractility and function, but at other times described a much vaguer general improvement of the "circulation." The Chinese scientists, physicians, and translators often appeared confused when trying to explain the traditional meaning of these phrases to what appeared to be uncomprehending foreigners. In contrast, however, in the physical sciences, less bound by historical traditions, there were no intrinsic differences in semantic values. In a way, therefore, the problems were similar to those encountered when we read the Western literature of earlier periods.

We could in retrospect have eased our quest by more diligent attempts, prior to our visit, to absorb the principles and theory of Chinese traditional medicine, difficult though it might have been. Yet we learned that even Western-trained <u>Chinese</u> physicians do not find it easy to master the traditional concepts and that all Chinese are limited in their comprehension because the bulk of traditional classics remain untranslated from the original archaic language in which they were written.

Nor was our lot made easier by our ignorance of Chinese patterns of disease.[7] Repeatedly, we learned that disease statistics in the United States and China differed radically. For instance, appendicitis occurs (or at least is diagnosed) quite commonly (in one hospital it constituted 10% of all surgical admissions). Yet it is seen infrequently in Chinese children, and is most common in male adults, whereas in the United States it is common in children and certainly does not spare females. With such differences, can one use "historical" controls from one culture to assess data from another? Is appendicitis the same disease in the two countries?[8] Are the differences real, or can they be explained by diagnostic prejudice, tradition, and error? What can one assume about the "natural history" of such a disease? What criteria do we employ to evaluate the putative amelioration seen in Chinese patients after treatment with remedies foreign to us?

The timing of our visit, not too long after the dislocations caused by the Cultural Revolution, also had an impact. It was beyond contention that the entire academic and research structure had been shaken, and there was abundant evidence that a new equilibrium may not yet have been reached, let alone a new optimal state. We met competent scientists who had been sent down to the countryside, with at least temporary derailment of their scientific careers, and we were often shown work of such vintage as to suggest a paucity of more recent scientific research.

This, coupled with a post-Antonioni* sensitivity to criticism, elicited in us, in turn, a sense of counter-paranoia as we began to suspect (at times unjustly) that failure to be shown something we had requested for the itinerary meant either that it did not exist or was judged by our hosts as likely to strike us as inferior. We were, for example, not successful in visiting psychiatric units or in getting much information about the drug treatment of psychiatric ailments, but both Norwegian and Finnish delegations have seen Chinese psychiatry in considerable detail (as reported in Scandinavian psychiatric journals).

Sometimes trouble arose out of cultural values and thinking habits that were antipodal. We were, for instance, often interested in trying to decide whether "proof" or "evidence" existed that one variable determined the fate of another. How, we speculated, could one be sure that an herb (or six to ten herbs, more often, perhaps changed every day or so) had <u>really</u> altered a patient's course? We were dissatisfied with the Chinese <u>post hoc, ergo propter hoc</u> attitude, which seemed happy with "improvement" and seemed to care little for assigning specific credit with precision.

Many Westerners are skeptical of traditional remedies; the Chinese repeatedly told us that remedies used by the people for centuries <u>must</u> be effective. Westerners have been trained in a type of pharmacologic puritanism, believing that a chemical capable of doing good must also be capable of doing harm (at least to some); to the Chinese, traditional remedies are universally proclaimed as safe, and they find no paradox in the ability of a chemical to alter bodily processes only in the direction of benefit. [Recent American experience with the traumatic and infectious complications of acupuncture suggests that the absence of Chinese concern in that area is perhaps unjustified.][9]

---

*The Italian filmmaker Antonioni's documentary on China is resented fiercely by the Chinese who feel that it overemphasizes the negative aspects of Chinese life.

We worship the placebo as an experimental "blank" or "control" while denigrating the purposeful "therapeutic" use of inert medications; the Chinese will not countenance the use of placebo controls, considering them to be unethical conceits, yet they accept the use of such remedies as ground pearl and rhinoceros horn, which sound suspiciously like placebos to the Western skeptic. A commentary in the JAMA of August 5, 1974 criticized the use of B-12 injections, saying "...it is better to select a completely inert placebo to avoid...confusion."[10] One suspects that the Chinese might question this approach, which seems to discount the therapeutic mileage to be gotten out of a faith by patient or doctor in the use of a placebo that at least carries the hope of pharmacologic effect above and beyond the psychological benefit.

Western science has made its greatest advances by isolating variables and purposely manipulating one while keeping others fixed (even at the price of artificiality). (Indeed, that is what a scientific experiment is, as opposed to an "experiment of nature.") The Chinese, on the other hand, seem quite unworried by the simultaneous application of several therapeutic modalities. It is all very well to say that the Chinese physician "tailors" his treatment to the individual, using clues found in the appearance of the patient's tongue or the feel of the radial pulse, but Western charlatans, quacks, and incompetents have said the same thing on too many occasions in the past for foreigners to rest easy when the Chinese physician authoritatively explains why his therapy is impossible to explain.

The Western physician or scientist also often has a natural tendency to view skeptically the use of crude plant or animal extracts as drugs. He forgets that many of our own useful drugs originated through an investigation of herbal medicines. Other misconceptions are that plant extracts are not used by physicians in the United States today and that most of our drugs originate from the synthetic chemist. Even a hasty look at the current status of botanicals and botanically derived drugs, however, should suffice to convince one that the United States still relies on plants as a major source of some of our most useful drugs.

A national survey of prescriptions dispensed from American community pharmacies during 1968 (hospital drugs were not considered) revealed that about 1.68 billion new and refilled prescriptions were dispensed. Of these prescriptions, 25 percent contained one or more active principles consisting of either (a) a crude plant material, (b) a crude extract obtained from plants, or (c) a purified active principle obtained from plants. Seventy-six pure active plant principles were found among these prescriptions, and all of them except seven (emetine, caffeine, theobromine, theophylline, pseudoephedrine, ephedrine, and papaverine) are still commercially extracted from plant materials (the seven listed above are produced by synthesis). Even more startling is the fact that 99 crude drugs, or crude extracts from plants, were encountered in the survey prescriptions. These crude drugs or extracts entering into the prescriptions were present in 41,451,000 prescriptions in 1968, or 2.5 percent of the total.

Listed below are the most important purified active principles from the plants revealed by the survey, together with the total number of prescriptions containing each ingredient and the percentage of total prescriptions for each ingredient.*

Active Plant Principle	Total Number of Rx	Percent of Total Rx
Codeine	34,060,000	2.03
Atropine	28,390,000	1.50
Reserpine	24,348,000	1.45
Pseudoephedrine	15,025,000	0.90
Ephedrine	13,003,000	0.77
Hyoscyamine	12,728,000	1.00
Digoxin	12,183,000	0.73
Scopolamine	11,453,000	0.66
Digitoxin	5,483,000	0.33
Pilocarpine	4,356,000	0.26
Quinidine	2,989,000	0.18

*Prescription survey data were kindly supplied by Dr. R.A. Gosselin, Massachusetts College of Pharmacy and analyzed by Dr. Norman R. Farnsworth, University of Illinois.

Also listed below are the most important crude botanical drugs or plant extracts that appeared in the survey.

Crude Botanical or Extract	Total Number of Rx	Percent of Total Rx
Belladonna (Atropa belladonna)	11,322,000	0.68
Opium (Papaver somniferum)	7,635,000	0.45
Rauwolfia (Rauvolfia serpentina)	6,307,000	0.38
Cascara (Rhamnus purshiana)	2,643,000	0.16
Digitalis (Digitalis purpurea)	2,636,000	0.16
Citrus bioflavonoids (Citrus sp.)	1,517,000	0.09
Veratrum (Veratrum viride)	1,188,000	0.07

Although this survey covers only those prescriptions dispensed from community pharmacies in the United States during 1968, a computerized analysis of similar data for the period 1959 through 1968 revealed that the percentages of these plant materials, as a function of the total number of prescriptions dispensed annually, remained approximately constant. It is presumed that plant materials used as drugs have not diminished in importance from 1968 up to the present time.

We were repeatedly puzzled by our failure to find students to talk to. Were they all harvesting crops? At Nanking we finally saw plenty of them (at the College of Pharmacy) but spoke to none. It was not until Canton that we finally got to talk to some; we were all impressed by their alertness and intelligence.

Another significant fact is that little personal contact was allowed between us and the Chinese scientists. We saw none of them on a one-to-one basis. We always spoke in groups; we went to no private homes. (It is apparently not Chinese tradition to entertain at home.) We had the impression that further interchange between ourselves and the Chinese scientists would be kept to a minimum, although we would be allowed to write to them at their hospital or university addresses. Our hosts were warm and polite, but, as if by unspoken agreement, any type of personal relationship was discouraged. The closest that anyone in our group could come to an interchange was conversations in the cars as we were driving in the cities. Here, however, we were monitored by the translator and other people in the car, and for most of us there was a considerable language barrier. Therefore, a main attribute of modern science - the personal friendship, correspondence, and intimate interchange between scientists seen so often in the West - was not a part of our visit.

THE WEDDING OF WESTERN AND TRADITIONAL MEDICINE

One of the most constantly reiterated principles on our Chinese trip was the need to combine the best elements of Western and Chinese traditional medicine. Mao Tse-tung has clearly been a major force in the struggle to raise traditional medicine to a higher level of recognition and respect from the Chinese medical establishment. We were constantly told, in our visits to various institutions, of Mao's statement that "Chinese traditional medicine and pharmacology are a great treasure house and vigorous efforts should be made to explore them and raise them to a higher level."

Today one sees a variegated picture as one visits different institutes and hospitals. All pay at least lip service to the need to fuse Western and traditional medicine. Some, however, seem to be predominantly Western in orientation, and some are at the other extreme. In certain institutions we gained the impression that the union of Western and Chinese medicine had not produced much strain between their separate practitioners. Other visits led to a different judgment. We found, for example, that some purely traditional institutes manifested a great deal of bitterness, within the context of the anti-Lin and anti-Confucius campaign, about their past status. The Cultural Revolution and its aftermath have given traditional Chinese physicians a new authority in medical work, and they naturally wish to preserve it.

Early in the trip, we visited the Institute of Chinese Materia Medica in Peking. The briefing we received was one of the most doctrinaire to be heard on the entire trip. The director of the Institute, with emotion and emphasis, gave us the most intense form of what might be called the current line on traditional Chinese medicine. As early as 1928, he asserted, Mao Tse-tung realized the importance of using traditional medicine, which was the product of two millennia of the Chinese people's struggle against disease. The Chairman has repeatedly stressed its importance, because reactionaries have been so eager to attack the virtues of Chinese medicine. During the nineteenth century, when China was "westernized," traitors and miscreants like Li Hung-chang tried to destroy this precious legacy. In the twentieth century it was also attacked by reactionaries like Yuan Shih-k'ai, Wang Ching-wei, Chiang Kai-shek, Liu Shao-ch'i, and Lin Piao. Fortunately, Chairman Mao was aware of the real motives of these latter-day "scoundrels and vipers" and therefore used the Great Proletarian Cultural Revolution and the current campaign to give Chinese medicine its proper due.

There was a fascinating mixture of elements in this argument: the nativism, the animus toward westernization, and the inconsistency (to us) in attacking Confucius while praising a traditional science. There is a long legacy of bitterness among traditional Chinese medical workers. Despite Mao Tse-tung's praise of traditional medicine in 1958, that sector, we were repeatedly told, had not been accorded much respect by the dominant Western-trained medical majority until the Cultural Revolution broke out. After the Cultural Revolution, the traditionalists had come back with a vengeance, drawing upon strong nativist feelings to defend their own claims. Nor was this feeling solely the director's. The Chinese technical workers around the table and the leading member of the Revolutionary Committee all showed approval as the director spoke in tones that were harsh and bore no hint of tolerance for other viewpoints.

A similar experience occurred 20 days later when we visited the Kwangtung College of Traditional Chinese Medicine in Canton. The same hard approach to the Liu-ist Line and an hour-long lecture by the vice-chairman of the Revolutionary Committee, followed by another lecture by vice-chairman of the Educational Revolutionary Committee, reflected the same tone we had heard in Peking.

In the institutes dominated by the best Western-style physicians, on the other hand, the mood was one of confidence, sometimes even accompanied by a certain amount of embarrassment over the terminology, concepts, and approach of the traditional Chinese medicine they now practiced. At the Tumor Prevention Research Institute near the old Legation Quarter in Peking, for example, the staff was composed of extremely competent doctors who were informed about latest Western techniques. Their questions about pharmaceutical preparations were very knowledgeable and there was no mistaking the high caliber of the personnel. At this institution, most of the treatment seemed to be Western.

There was more evidence of a fusion of styles at the Fu-wai Hospital in Peking. There we were shown cases of treatment with Chinese drugs for angina pectoris and shock and with acupuncture for high blood pressure and strokes. Pain was apparently reduced, and patients partially recovered the use of paralyzed limbs - though recovery in these cases (where the patient's psychological state is so crucial) may have been as much a matter of the staff's conscientious care and concern for the patient as the acupuncture _per se_. The union of Western and Chinese medicine seemed easier in an originally Western-style clinic like Fu-wai than in some of the other traditional medical institutes. The Western-style physicians here seemd much more willing to use the traditionalists' methods than _vice versa_. Perhaps because they are overcompensating for their lower status in the past, traditional Chinese doctors often appeared to be less willing to be eclectic, holding to their own techniques as purists would. (This could be simply a matter of training. It may be easier for a Western-style doctor to learn some traditional methods than the other way around.)

One way of dealing with the conflicts between Western and traditional medicines is to become totally eclectic. Fu-wai doctors may be electic, but they are not syncretic. Chinese drugs are prescribed according to ancient diagnostic methods for which the patient's tongue and pulse remain the most important indicators, none of which is readily translatable into Western terms. Eclecticism certainly achieves results, but one wonders how long the loose combination will continue to satisfy researchers on either side of the split. Western and Chinese medical theoretical structures exist side by side, compartmentalized. Doctors call upon one or the other according to the needs of the patient. But if theory is required, it may prove impossible to combine the two into a syncretic system to account for the efficacy of a given medical cure. The Western-style units are succeeding best at following the middle line of political and technical synthesis that Chairman Mao advocates, and yet it is precisely these units that are the most eclectic, the most contradictory in certain senses, about the ultimate scientific marriage of traditional and Western methods.

The word "traditional" medicine was used in a very broad sense, and it was not always clear how genuine the appellation was. It was applied not only to folk medicines, but to techniques used in special surgery. In Peking, for example, we saw some highly expert cataract surgery that looked thoroughly "modern," but were told that the site of scleral incision and a method called "couching" had been used centuries ago by Chinese surgeons. (The little plastic scoop for "netting" the cataract was quite new, however.)

In both Tientsin and Shanghai we saw remarkable results with a noncast approach to bone fractures. Broken bones are often set and simply splinted without immobilization of adjacent joints. The resultant early motion that is both possible and encouraged is said to improve the circulation and thus accelerate healing, and to avoid the stiffness and "freezing" so often seen after plaster cast immobilization. In Shanghai, some ingenious (and highly nontraditional!) plastic hinged splints had been developed as adjuvants.

How much of this clever orthopedic approach is really "traditional"? We were told that peasants treated bone fractures in this way, which seems perfectly reasonable, since plaster of paris is not available to them, but one wonders whether some bright orthopedist didn't just think of trying this 10 to 15 years ago, and whether the relation to "tradition" isn't a generous (or astute) concession to the popular party line. [A recent letter to the editor of the British Medical Journal of 22 June, 1974, says: "Dr. Smith would have been equally impressed if he had visited St. Peter's Hospital in Chertsey, where fractured femurs are initially treated in identical fashion. It makes me wonder whether in fact Chinese treatment is really St. Peter's treatment and whether, perhaps, Chairman Mao paid us a surreptitious visit before the cultural revolution (or *vice versa*?)."]

Acupuncture analgesia, which is much more impressive and convincing than therapeutic acupuncture, is also a hard technique to pigeonhole. Acupuncture was not used for surgical anesthesia prior to 15 years ago. The points of stimulation are more empiric than "traditional," and the electric current applied to the needles is certainly "Western." To what extent, then, is acupuncture analgesia "traditional"?

Despite the political popularity of traditional medicine, Western medicine still seems to be in the ascendancy. Most physicians being turned out in 1974 were apparently enrolled in Western-style schools. At one traditional school we were told that the percentage of female students was 25 percent (20 percent is "required"), whereas in a Western-type school we found 50 percent of students to be women - not much of a female testimonial for tradition!

THE CLINICAL USE OF HERBAL MEDICINES*

The genesis of interest in herbal drugs lies in their perceived clinical benefits. The philosophic concepts of ancient Chinese medicine are closely intermeshed with such usage, but for both the masses and the scientific-medical establishment, it is the empiric performance of these natural products that provides the basis for their use and for research. Before discussing the laboratory explorations of traditional medicines, it seems logical to describe what we saw in the way of their clinical usage and the benefits ascribed to them.

Treatment of Acute Abdominal Conditions by Nonsurgical Means

This general subject is a major one in modern Chinese medicine and is a good example of how traditional and Western medicine are combined. Perhaps the best example of this was seen in the Nan K'ai Hospital in Tientsin, where an acute abdominal conditions research group, very active in a variety of diseases of this type, have published several reports of their work in the Chinese Medical Journal. Four types of acute abdominal conditions treated by this group were described for us: appendicitis, perforated ulcer, acute pancreatitis, and common duct stones. All these conditions are treated with one or more of the following: acupuncture, Chinese herbs, and Western-style medical care. The data on appendicitis are particularly illustrative.

According to discussions with the Nan K'ai group and their short publication in the Chinese Medical Journal[1], 995 cases had been treated nonoperatively from 1963 to 1972. Of these, 93.6 percent is the percentage given for uneventful recovery for simple acute appendicitis. If there was suppuration, the success rate decreased to 76 percent; when there was peritonitis, the rate was 50 percent. The treatment is a combination of certain herb medicines to promote the blood circulation and, occasionally, aspiration of the abscesses.

Further intensive discussion of acute appendicitis was carried out in Shanghai, at the Lung Hua Hospital of Traditional Medicine, which is also associated with a general teaching hospital. Here, again, we saw cases of

---

*The term "herbal medicines" is used here to cover medicaments from a variety of natural sources. Plants constitute the major source of these natural products; animals and minerals are minor sources.

acute appendicitis that were treated with traditional drugs. We were told that there is no word for acute appendicitis in traditonal Chinese medicine; it is known as an abdominal abscess and was classically treated with herbal medicines as far back as the fifth century. We were told that since the Cultural Revolution there have been as many as 20,000 cases of appendicitis treated in China with herbal drugs, with a 90 percent overall cure rate. In this hospital 364 cases of nonsurgical approach to simple, nonperforated appendicitis have been reviewed. The average time for cure was 3½ days. We were told that 30 percent of the patients with appendicitis ultimately undergo operation. If peritonitis sets in, surgery and Western antibiotics such as penicillin and streptomycin are used.

We observed that the prescription used for the treatment of acute appendicitis varied from hospital to hospital in China. Some examples of the various mixtures, together with an explanation of the pharmacologic effects reported in the literature for the various plant components, are given below.

Rx *Rheum tanguticum*

Magnolia officinalis

Taraxacum mongolicum

Sargentodoxa cuneata

Rx *Rheum tanguticum*

Magnolia officinalis

Sonchus bracyotus

Sargentodoxa cuneata

Rx *Rheum tanguticum*

Taraxacum mongolicum

Lonicera japonica

Prunus persica

Paeonia lactiflora

Akebia guinata

Corydalis bulbosa

Prunus mume

Talc

An untranslatable ingredient

Rheum tanguticum is the only ingredient common to the three prescriptions, and it could exert a laxative effect due to the anthraquinones known to be present in this plant. In addition, the anthraquinones may contribute an antibacterial effect. Nothing is reported in the scientific literature relative to the pharmacological effects of *Magnolia* species that would explain its inclusion in the prescription. Certain *Magnolia* species do contain cytotoxic sesquiterpene lactones, which might be predicted to have antimicrobial effects. Pharmacological effects have not been published for *Taraxacum mongolicum*, but the related *Taraxacum officinale* has shown antibacterial properties. *Lonicera japonica* extracts have also shown *in vitro* antibacterial effects, as have extracts of *Prunus mume*. *Paeonia lactiflora* has not been investigated pharmacologically, but paeoniflorin has been isolated from the related *Paeonia suffruticosa*, and has shown anti-inflammatory and antipyretic properties in animals. *Paeonia moutan* extracts have also shown *in vitro* antibacterial activity, as well as antipyretic activity in animals.

The stated rationale for these mixtures by Chinese medical doctors was to evacuate the intestine (an approach contrary to Western teaching, where cathartics are contraindicated in acute appendicitis), achieve antibacterial effects, and promote circulation to the damaged organ. All three prescriptions might satisfy the first two criteria, but data are lacking to support the thesis that any of the plants promotes circulation.

Other abdominal emergencies treated at Nan K'ai by nonoperative procedures included perforated ulcer, pancreatitis, and common duct stone. All three were treated with a combination of acupuncture and Chinese herbs that are stated to be anti-inflammatory. A paper has appeared on their ulcer series of 316 cases, of which 69 percent were treated nonoperatively and 31 percent surgically.[2] This article lists four different herb preparations that are used in addition to acupuncture. One of these is said to reduce the volume and acidity of gastric secretion; another appears to promote intestinal peristalsis; still another is considered effective in improving circulation; and the last appears to inhibit the growth of organisms in the intestinal tract and also "detoxifies the endotoxin of *S. typhosa*." In the Nan K'ai Hospital in Tientsin, considerable research on animals is being pursued to validate these ideas. These studies include the ability of either drugs or acupuncture to induce phagocytosis and to reduce experimental inflammation. There was a close connection in the Nan K'ai Hospital between experimental work and the surgical problems that were encountered in the wards.

We also saw a number of patients, both in Tientsin and in the Peking Municipal Hospital of Chinese Traditional Medicine, in whom nonsurgical, herbal treatment was used for kidney stones and gallstones. The Chinese are particularly proud of nonsurgical treatment for both of these. The drug treatment is extremely complicated and combines herbal drugs with such Western standards as morphine, atropine, and magnesium sulfate. This is now their routine approach to the treatment of both types of stones, but again a critical evaluation of either the pharmacology involved or the actual statistics appears to be lacking.

While nonsurgical treatment of some of these conditions seems strange to Westerners, it should be remembered that similar approaches have been utilized in such situations as appendicitis on a small ship lacking a surgeon, or perforated ulcer in U.S. soldiers during World War II. The limited experience suggested that such nonsurgical treatment at the very least is not necessarily disastrous. We, too, are now studying the use of a nonsurgical approach, chenodeoxycholic acid, to dissolve gallstones in vivo.

Arthritic Disorders

We saw, in the Kiangsu Provincial Hospital of Chinese Traditional Medicine in Nanking, a 42-year-old woman with a history of sore throat about 3 weeks previously, who was admitted with polyarthritis several days before our arrival. This disease was presumably acute rheumatic fever. This woman and others like her with either rheumatic fever or rheumatoid arthritis are apparently rarely treated with aspirin. Continued questions about this point led to the answer that aspirin was too toxic and that the Chinese did not get good results with it, so they used traditional herbs, which allegedly helped the symptoms and decreased the sedimentation rate. It is possible that these herbs, like salicylates (which, after all, were originally derived from plants) have an anti-inflammatory effect;* research is going on in this area. A similar discussion about rheumatoid arthritis and a review of several patients occurred in the Municipal Hospital in Tientsin in connection with their orthopedic program.

---

*Many plant constituents have been reported in the world literature to produce anti-inflammatory effects in animal models. These include the alkaloids holaphylline, dregamine, gentianine, gentianidine, ephedrine, taspine, abrine, chaksine, cytisine, lupinine, sparteine, colchicine, colchicoside, edpetiline, petiline, cryogenine, tomatine, sinomenine, isotetrandrine, tetrandrine, damascenine, thalsimine, dihydrothalsimine, thalfoetidine, thalmine, O-methylthalicberine, thalcimine, dihydrothalcimine, thalictrinine, fetidine, emetine, scopolamine, solasodine, tuberosine, badchysine, cycleanine, dauricine, nuciferine, carnosine and homocarnosine; the flavonoids rutin, quercetin, hyperoside, luteolin, luteolin-7-glucoside, liquiritin, liquiritigenin, licurizid, liquiritone, isoliquiritin, neoliquiritin, taxifolin, isoliquiritigenin, neoisoliquiritin, leucodelphinidin, kaempferol, kaempferitrin, kaempferol-7-glucoside, kaempferol-3-O-arabinoside, kaempferol-3-O-rhamnofuranoside; the steroidal sapogenins diosgenin, cryptogenin, and ruscogenin; the triterpenes and triterpene glycosides Panax saponin A, gypsogenin glycoside, cycloartanol, 24-methylenecycloartanol, cyclosadol, citrostadienol, aescin, alpha aescin, cryptoaescin, japokryptoaescin B, tectorigenin, tectoridin, oleanolic acid glycoside, glycyrrhetinic acid, glycyrrhetic acid, liquiritic acid, glycyrrhizin; and the miscellaneous plant products curcumin, zygophyllin, quinovic acid, the saikosides, imperatorin, heraclenin, ternoside, paeoniflorin, esculin, aesculetin, paeonol, jaligonic acid, kawain, dihydrokawain, methysticin, dihydromethysticin, yangonin, desmethoxyyangonin, azulene, fraxin, allisatin, acacetin, coumarin, an en-yne dicycloether, and (-)-alpha-bisabolol.

Orthopedics

Although herbal pharmacology was involved hardly at all in these patients, they are included because we spent two half-days in excellent orthopedic hospitals reviewing the nonsurgical treatment of various orthopedic problems and emergencies. The first was the Municipal Hospital in Tientsin, which specializes in the closed, nonsurgical reduction of broken bones.

After seeing a movie explaining the technique, we were taken to an operating room where a 14-year-old schoolgirl lay on a table with both bones of her right forearm broken from an accident during physical exercise. When we entered the operating room, she had been undergoing acupuncture for 20 minutes from two electrically stimulated needles in her arm. Without giving her any other anesthesia, two doctors pulled her arm, stretching the bones apart at the fracture site, while a third doctor molded the bones into place with an audible click. Although the patient had a fixed smile on her face throughout, she winced once, during the most extreme point of the reduction. Short splints were applied immediately and tied with bandages, and just as soon as that was done the patient was asked to start exercising her hand. We were told that she would be released shortly afterward to return home.

An astonishing part of our morning visit was seeing two women who had been injured in bicycle accidents. Their x-rays indicated compression fractures of the lower spine. Yet instead of being placed in a body cast, they had been taught how to do "bridging" exercises in their beds while their spines healed. The Chinese doctors discussed the form and rate of exercise with each patient, which presumably gives a considerable sense of self-confidence to the invalids. By their own efforts and will (again, Mao's thought is stressed), they were effecting their own cures. "We let each patient cure himself," the orthopedist explained.

In Shanghai we saw a second excellent orthopedic unit, this time at the Jui Chin Hospital, which is the teaching hospital for the Second Shanghai Medical School. Here again they specialize in closed reduction with an avoidance, in general, of plaster casts. The method of splinting was different in the two hospitals; particularly ingenious splints made of curved and hinged plastic are used in the Shanghai Hospital. The impressive director of the orthopedic unit in Shanghai, Chien Pu-fan, spoke good English but had not been abroad. He has been director of this unit for 13 years.

Orthopedics in China thus shows the vitality of clinical medicine there along practical lines, eliminating what may be unnecessary operative interference and making the treatment of disease simple, so as to return ill workers as quickly as possible to their jobs and to develop techniques that can be readily applied in the countryside. All this is done without any obvious sacrifice of good medical treatment or postoperative care. (It should be added that in some orthopedic situations, such as congenital hip dislocation, the Chinese use Western methods exclusively.)

Cancer

We saw cancer patients at the Cancer Institute associated with the Jih Tan Hospital in Peking, also called the Municipal Tumor Hospital, and at the

Capital Hospital in Peking (the former Peking Union Medical College). In general, herbal medicines were not used for the treatment of cancer, but the treatment of tumors in both places does shed some light on the balance that is being struck between Western and traditional medicine in China. The Cancer Institute was founded in 1958. This relatively late date is explained by the fact that contagious diseases had been considered the main health problem at the time of Liberation. Although cancer was only ninth on the mortality list in 1951, in some parts of China it is now first or second, and great efforts are being made to control it. Because the government recognizes that it is a high-incidence disease, the hospital across the street, which was part of the Institute, is soon to be expanded. In the meantime, as part of the Cultural Revolution, the Institute's doctors are making greater efforts to focus on specific forms of cancer that have unusually high rates of occurrence in specific regions of China: nasopharyngeal cancer in the South, liver cancer in the East, and esophageal forms in the North. Throughout the country, special coordinating groups have been established to attack these diseases, and this Institute has conducted a cytologic-smear survey of 50 million people in three provinces of central and northern China. Certain districts in western Anhwei were thereby discovered to have an extraordinarily high rate of cancer of the throat, and special research teams were subsequently sent to those areas. This permitted detection of the disease much earlier, bringing the 5-year survival rate up to 70-80 percent.

Some interesting correlations were discovered. For example, those areas with a high prevalence of esophageal cancer also had a high incidence of gullet cancer in chickens, with the same histology seen in humans (squamous cell carcinoma). Research is now being conducted to explain this fascinating correlation with particular emphasis on carcinogens (such as nitrosamine) in food or water. The doctors used traditional Chinese medicines only as supportive treatment (and with a minimum of clinically significant effect). Indeed, they relied mainly on early detection, radiology, and expert surgery (their esophageal cancer patients' mortality rate under surgery was only 1.4 percent) to combat this disease, and they do not emphasize drugs of either Western or Chinese origin in its treatment.

With respect to treatment of tumors generally, the group at the Jih Tan Hospital seem completely aware of modern chemotherapeutic methods.

In the Capital Hospital at Peking, we were shown patients from their series on the chemotherapy of choriocarcinoma, a more common disease in China than in the United States. Since 1958, the gynecologists in this hospital have treated 800 cases of metastatic choriocarcinoma, using not the standard Western drugs (methotrexate and *Vinca* alkaloids), but a combination of 5-fluorouracil and 6-mercaptopurine. We were told the dosage schedule and given detailed accounts of the courses of various patients, as well as the statistics involved. The staff appeared competent and is achieving highly satisfactory results in the majority of patients. They claim that the two drugs that they are using are less toxic than the ones being used in the West. Nothing was said in any of these conversations about herbal remedies. [Both here and in other situations, it appears that when there are existing efficacious Western drugs for serious illness, herbal remedies are often either not used or are only added to existing regimens in a "supportive" way, at least in Western-type hospitals. This is significant for two reasons: (1) it shows that good medical care is not necessarily compromised, even with the tremendous political pressure to utilize "traditional medicine," and (2) it is difficult to evaluate herbal medicines when they are being used in combination with effective Western drugs.]

At the Capital Hospital we also saw several cases of lung cancer, which seems less common in China than in the West. Squamous cell carcinoma accounts for only 40 percent of lung cancers in China, whereas it accounts for about 90 percent in the West. As many Westerners have observed, Chinese smoke a great deal; perhaps cigarette smoking is not prohibited or proscribed in China because the Chinese are less susceptible to lung cancer than we are, although the incidence there is said to be increasing, and the estimated lag period is such that the full impact of the smoking may not yet be apparent. (Another possibility is that Chinese inhale cigarette smoke less than Westerners do; we certainly had this impression.)

The patients were being treated vigorously with a combination of radiotherapy, actinomycin D, and 5-fluorouracil. We were told that the treatment was successful in several of these patients and that the various types of carcinoma responded differentially to drugs (adenocarcinoma best, squamous (cell least). As a general aside to this discussion of cancer in both the Capital Hospital and Jih Tan Hospital, the care of all the patients we saw appeared excellent, with an imaginative and aggressive approach to chemotherapy.

Infectious Diseases

We did not see many cases of infectious diseases. One woman with erysipelas, who was recovering, had not been given antibiotics, but only local treatment, because of "sensitivity to antibiotics." She had received local applications of herbs in a plaster but no systemic drugs.

Later we saw an interesting patient in our visit to the Kiangsu Provincial Hospital of Chinese Traditional Medicine in Nanking, where much traditional treatment is used, including moxibustion and acupuncture. An 18-year-old girl with pneumococcal pneumonia had been admitted 10 days earlier with classical symptoms of that disease and one lobe affected. She was not treated with penicillin but with herbal remedies. (The herbal prescription for pneumococcal pneumonia was composed of the following plants:

Rx _Polygonum cymosum_

Houttuynia cordata

Ajuga decumbens

_Prunella vulgaris_*

The only rational basis for the use of this mixture, according to literature reports, is that the anthraquinones predicted to be present in _Polygonum cymosum_ might have antimicrobial activity.)

---

*Erroneously indicated throughout the trip as _Brunella vulgaris_.

We asked about other infectious diseases, such as meningitis, and were told that there was not much meningitis in China. (We learned, however, that the herbal treatment for meningitis was composed of the following ingredients:

Rx *Anemarrhena asphodeloides*

Glycyrrhiza uralensis

White tiger broth

Gypsum

There is no rational basis for the use of this mixture for meningitis according to presently available literature reports on the chemical constituents or pharmacological activities of the components.)

In the discussion the important point was made that a principle of traditional medicine was not simply to treat the infection or attack the bacteria, but to treat the "whole patient." We surmised that at this institution, drugs such as penicillin and streptomycin were used only in severe infections.

We tried on several occasions to find out whether the Chinese had a significant problem with allergy or idiosyncrasy to penicillin, but never got a satisfactory answer. It is interesting, however, that penicillin is one of the few drugs that was said to require a prescription for purchase. In the drugstores in the city, virtually all drugs are freely available, except for the narcotics. Sulfonamides, isoniazid, and the tetracyclines were available without prescription, as were such drugs as chlordiazepoxide, diazepam, meprobamate, and acetazolamide. Chloramphenicol is apparently used with frequency and presumably produces the expected incidence of aplastic anemia, but we had no personal opportunity to look into this aspect of the relatively free access of Chinese to drugs of all kinds.

Cardiovascular Diseases

We saw patients with cardiovascular diseases at a number of hospitals, beginning with the Fu Wai Hospital in Peking and including the Capital Hospital in Peking and the Jui Chin Hospital in Shanghai. Cases of angina, myocardial infarction, and congestive heart failure were shown to us. The general pattern was the same throughout, with patients getting excellent care by Western standards. The ones with failure were digitalized and treated with Western diuretics. We saw a few cases of hypertension being treated with reserpine and hydrochlorothiazide. We also saw outpatients in some of the traditional hospitals who had suffered strokes and were coming back for acupuncture treatment.

However, treatment in this important class of diseases is often overlaid with the use of herbal medicine. One herbal preparation being used for myocardial infarction and anginal pain was administered intravenously in ampul form and consisted of an aqueous extract of the following:

Rx *Salvia miltiorhiza*

Dalbergia odorifera

There is no direct evidence in the literature that either of the plants in this prescription would be effective in the management of myocardial infarction or anginal pain. However, the volatile oil from other *Salvia* species has been shown to produce hypotension in laboratory animals, and ursolic acid, a triterpene present in most *Salvia* species, has been shown to be a diuretic in animals.

We visited a pharmacology laboratory where this preparation was being administered intravenously to an anesthetized dog, whose blood pressure and cardiac output were being recorded. The experiment had been in progress for some time, and it appeared that the herbal preparation had decreased blood pressure by approximately 50 percent, with a duration in excess of 3 hours. Also, cardiac output was increased by about 50 percent. These observations suggest that the plants in this mixture should be further investigated with a view to isolation of the active principle(s).

Another herbal prescription being used orally for hypertension and to increase a low hemoglobin count consisted of the following ingredients:

Rx *Scutellaria baicalensis*

Codonopsis pilosula

Ligusticum wallichii

Spatholobus suberectus

Paeonia obovata

Carthamus tinctorius

Piper longum

Asarum heterotropoides var. *mandshuricum*

Citrus sinensis (peel)

Alpinia officinarum

Pistacia lentiscus

Trichosanthes kirilowii

Extracts of *Scutellaria baicalensis* have been shown to elicit diuretic, cardiotonic, and sedative effects in laboratory animals. Although *Paeonia obovata* has not been investigated, *Paeonia suffruticosa* has yielded paeoniflorin, which has shown anti-inflammatory and hypotensive activity in animals.

Species of Asarum other than the one indicated in the prescription have shown sedative activity in animals. Although controversial, the citrus bioflavonoids (Citrus sinensis peel) have long been alleged by some to decrease capillary fragility. Finally, extracts of Codonopsis pilosula have been reported to increase the red blood cell count in rats by 17.5 percent over controls. Thus, there exists some experimental justification for the use of this complex prescription for the conditions indicated, although the active crystalline components are largely unknown.

We had occasion to discuss herbal medicine with Wu Ying-k'ai, head of the Fu Wai Hospital in Peking, and his staff. Wu is a surgeon who originally trained at the Peking Union Medical College and then spent several years in Evarts Graham's Department of Surgery at Washington University in St. Louis. It was our impression that some of the physicians (most of them Western-trained) believe that some interesting results have been obtained with herbal medicine, which is in the trial-and-error stage. There is no unwillingness on their part to try herbal medicine, so long as it does not hurt anybody. Neither patient care nor research was being compromised in any way by the use of herbs. In addition to the herbal remedies that occasionally are used in the treatment of cardiovascular disease, patients often receive therapeutic acupuncture. This is common practice following stroke or myocardial infarction. We saw a woman of 44 years, who had severe hypertensive disease culminating in stroke, with acupuncture needles in her face as well as several down the paralyzed side of her body. The "dosage schedule" for acupuncture consists of only about 30 minutes every other day (hardly an overwhelming "dose"!).

We saw a serious attempt to evaluate herbal drugs and acupuncture in angina at the Fu Wai Hospital, which included monitoring symptoms, electrocardiograms, and the appearance and the disappearance of radioactive iodinated serum albumin over the heart as a measure of cardiac blood flow. Data on 100 patients had been compiled but there appeared relatively little difference between pretreatment and posttreatment values. (Mao Tse-tung's teaching does in fact favor the experimental method, and part of the Cultural Revolution was alleged to be a questioning of established ideas. One can find in Mao's writing, over and over again, the injunction to reject classical ideas as they are taught and to use the experimental method to be self-reliant and to strike out on one's own.)

Neurological Diseases

Most of the patients with neurological diseases were seen at the excellent Hua Shan Hospital, which is the teaching hospital of the First Medical College in Shanghai. We saw patients with familial cerebellar ataxia, ascending spinal myelitis, and stroke and talked about epilepsy and multiple sclerosis.

In general, the neurological diseases of the "incurable" type are treated with both acupuncture and herbal medicine, but we could not really evaluate the efficacy of treatment. The same is true of cases of hemiplegia following stroke; again, acupuncture is used in addition to mixtures of herbal remedies. Amyotrophic lateral sclerosis apparently responds only minimally to traditional drugs. In the case of epilepsy, diphenylhydantoin is used, but herbal medicines are also employed.

In the Traditional Hospital in Peking we saw an outpatient with Bell's palsy who was being treated with a half hour of acupuncture every other day.

Burn Unit

We visited a remarkable burn unit at the Jui Chin Hospital in Shanghai. There we saw wards and private rooms with about 20 patients recovering from third-degree burns, in some cases over more than 90 percent of body surface. Some of these unfortunate men had fallen into lime pits; others had been burned in gasoline fires. We were given various statistics of their recovery from these severe burns; these percentages seemed better than those achieved in the West. General procedures in taking care of these people were outlined, and they appeared similar to Western techniques. Relatively little was said about herbal drugs except that "plasters" were routinely used at one point in the course and then removed at the time that the eschar is separated from the body.

Eye Diseases

Several of us visited the Eye Hospital affiliated with Chung Shan Medical College in Canton. We had discussion with three well-trained ophthalmologists, Chou Wen-ping, Tu Nien-tzu, and Hsia Fei, who were well conversant with principles of Western treatment but continually interpolated ideas of traditional medicine into the discussion as well. The first disease to be discussed was retinitis pigmentosa. It was mentioned that according to traditional Chinese teaching this eye disease arises from a weakness in the kidney. In the treatment of retinitis pigmentosa, the important element was to "warm up the kidney and raise the level of yang." For this they use a decoction of eight drugs in conjunction with an acupuncture regimen involving the application of a concentrated salt solution. Moxibustion was used as well. In a series of 144 patients, the ophthalmologists claimed that they improved the sight in 73 percent of them and that dark adaptation was improved in 62 percent.

The next discussion concerned uveitis, for which they gave intramuscular injections of a drug from an *Ilex* species and also a substance called *mao tun ch'ing*. It was stated that uveitis was caused in part by "internal heat in the liver" and that by use of these various traditional medicines, 60 percent of the patients were helped. Traumatic hyphema was treated in the same way.

The next disease to be discussed was viral keratitis. The Chinese acknowledge the usefulness of idoxuridine for the treatment of viral keratitis but said that it did not always work. (Their experiences with this drug seem to have been similar to those in the West, where it is now well known that a reasonable proportion of cases are not permanently cured by this drug and that there are frequent relapses.) The Chinese solution is to add herbal medicines to idoxuridine; this combination, they implied, yields better results.

Finally, we discussed glaucoma. For closed-angle glaucoma they use a combination of Chinese and Western medicine (such as drops of pilocarpine, 1 or 2 percent, together with oral acetazolamide, 250 mg every 6 or 8 hours).

We were then told about the etiology of glaucoma according to traditional medicine: There is a belief that "the liver opens the eye"; therefore they give a decoction (called Hsieh-Kan-San) that "promotes the flow of bile." Hsieh-Kan-San is composed of the following ingredients:

Rx *Rheum tanguticum*

Scutellaria baicalensis

Anemarrhena asphodeloides

Gentiana scabra

Scrophularia ningpoensis

Plantago asiatica

Zingiber officinalis

Angelica sinensis

Sodium sulfate

This prescription would have the following pharmacological activities, based on current knowledge of the constituents of the plants indicated or on reports of the activity in animals of crude extracts of the plants: The *Rheum tanguticum* would exert a cathartic effect due to the presence of anthraquinones, which could also contribute some antimicrobial activity. Gentianine, an alkaloid with established anti-inflammatory activity in animal models, is present in *Gentiana scabra*. *Scutellaria baicalensis* has been shown to exert diuretic effects in animals, and the diuretic principles wogonin, baicalin, and baicalein (all flavonoids) have been isolated from this plant. *Anemarrhena asphodeloides* has shown hypoglycemic activity in rabbits, and the steroidal saponins present in this plant would be predicted to have anti-inflammatory activity. Finally, *Plantago asiatica* extracts have shown diuretic activity in animals, and the related plant *Plantago ovata* has been reported to possess cholinergic activity.

For open-angle glaucoma, the Western treatment and that used by the Chinese is the same, pilocarpine plus acetazolamide and sometimes epinephrine also. However, to this is added acupuncture. We saw a patient who had come in a few days before with an intraocular pressure of 40 mm Hg; the pilocarpine and acetazolamide combination did not reduce it very much. He then was given acupuncture every day in the shoulder muscle, and the pressure had dropped to normal (20 mm Hg) by the time of our visit.

The treatment of eye diseases illustrates the degree to which traditional medicine is being incorporated into treatment in China, even by physicians who are trained primarily in the Western way. It also illustrates the enormous difficulty in making any evaluations of these herbal drugs. The drugs are exceedingly complex mixtures; they may not even be the same ones from day to day; there is no guarantee that they are prepared in precisely the same manner.

A decoction of eight plants could contain literally hundreds of different chemicals. Finally, careful records and controls usually are not kept, although a few groups are attempting to evaluate the overall results (illustrated here in the cases of retinitis pigmentosa and uveitis). However, serious attempts to quantify treatment effects against knowledge of the course of the untreated disease or to evaluate herbal medicine with and without Western medicine seem lacking.

Conclusions

A formidable barrier to identifying unequivocally effective elements from the field of herbal pharmacology is that there are so few clinical situations controlled enough to permit a positive statement. The problem is precisely that described by Bonica[3] with respect to therapeutic acupuncture. Herbal decoctions are widely used in connection with Western drugs, and are often used in chronic diseases (such as degenerative neurological disorders or chronic angina or long-term recovery from stroke) where prognosis and critical evaluation are exceedingly difficult. On the positive side, it must be stated that patients in China seem to do as well as those in the West at the hospitals we visited, and the present amalgam of Chinese and Western medicine may be as good as (or better than) any other system that might be devised for the Chinese population. Furthermore, the "marriage" of the two systems _is_ moving ahead without obvious dislocation - e.g., the chiefs of service in the hospitals seem to be trained in both. Nor did we really hear any criticism of Western medicine _per se_.

Nevertheless, many Western scientists, with their background and bias, will be troubled by traditional medicine, much of which represents a throwback to an earlier day in which the germ theory of disease and the etiology of many noninfectious diseases were unknown. Little of traditional medicine is being subjected to scientific proof or even to semicritical scrutiny, and we saw cases in which patients may not have received the best treatment by Western standards. (It is interesting that the same point has just been made strongly by Robert Hsu in connection with drug administration by barefoot doctors.[4]) Three examples can be cited: the case of pneumonia that was not given penicillin or any other antibiotics, the case of erysipelas that was not given any antibiotic, and a case of acute rheumatic fever for whom the plans following discharge from the hospital did not include long-term prophylactic use of either a sulfonamide or penicillin. Clearly, this is arguing from our own therapeutic habits, but the scientific and clinical basis for the management of these three diseases is such that one is perhaps entitled to be somewhat critical of the treatment.

In defense of the approaches employed by the Chinese, we were told that traditional medicine treats the whole patient and that the elimination of bacteria, for example, is secondary. (This presumably explains why 6-Hydroxyatropine is said to be effective in meningitis. There is a complex theory in Chinese medicine regarding blood flow and the increase of volume and flow in treating certain diseases; we heard this theory several times in connection with possible mechanisms of action of plant remedies as well.)

Having expressed these concerns, one must admit that certain of the practices now being used in China challenged our beliefs in a fascinating and potentially productive way. Among these were the nonoperative treatment of appendicitis, new approaches to cataract surgery, and the avoidance of plaster cast immobilization in orthopedics. It should be noted, however, that all of these examples do not necessarily involve herbal medicine, and, indeed, in the case of the orthopedic and ophthalmologic practices, the success of the method is in no way dependent on herbal drugs.

The conflict in theoretical background was brought home by a discussion of psychiatric and neurological theory and treatment in traditional medicine at the Kiangsu College of New Medicine in Nanking. We were told about the traditional theory of the causes of mania which are related to the "backing up of sputum," although by "sputum" they mean something analogous to our medieval "humors." (Indeed, there is unquestionable parallelism between their system of "sputum," "wind" and "fire" and the medieval Western theory of humors.)

They also made the point that Parkinson's disease is caused by "an excess of wind." In traditional medicine this is treated with acupuncture, although in the Western-type Hua Shan Hospital in Shanghai they seemed quite familiar with the use of L-dopa. This conversation at Nanking made us realize once again that the training and the philosophy of traditional and Western physicians are not at all close. It was also clear that a very real mandate has been given by Chairman Mao to medical workers in China to marry traditional and Western medicine. In further conversations with our hosts, they said that the ultimate (and far-off) goal is to produce a unified system of medicine incorporating both traditional and Western methods.

We might still ask the important question: Why traditional medicine? How did it arise and become such a powerful driving force in the wake of Liberation and then, even more so, in the wake of the Cultural Revolution? In Martin Cherkasky's report from the medical delegation that visited the People's Republic of China, June 15 to July 6, 1973,[5] he explains that there was no other way in which China could operate its health care program: "The decision to base a very large part of medicine in China today on traditional medicine and to insist upon the combining of Western and traditional medicine was the only sound policy that China could adopt." But Cherkasky seems to have confused traditional medicine with the whole scheme of paraprofessional medical care and barefoot doctors. The training of a traditional doctor at present is at least as difficult and takes at least as much time as the training of a Western physician. It is probably sound policy for China to reduce the medical curriculum, to integrate certain courses, and to delete others that may be of peripheral importance to the practice of medicine, but this has little to do with the establishment of traditional medicine as a major part of training and practice.

The push for traditional medicine may lie less in enlightened empiricism than deep at the heart of Chairman Mao's own personality, his romantic vision of the past, his rural origins, and his tremendous concern with the masses (and particularly the peasants) of China. Traditional medicine fits into this way of thinking about the past and present. Mao and other political leaders will of necessity lack technical knowledge of the deficiencies (or even of the balance of deficiencies and assets) in the enormously complex edifice of religion, philosophy, psychology, pharmacognosy, acupuncture, and the numerous other components that are traditional medicine.

CHINESE PHARMACOLOGY

Relative to other biologic sciences, pharmacology occupies an exalted position in the People's Republic of China, where the emphasis given to pharmacology is greater than in many other countries. This distinction is, however, perhaps more the result of political action than of scientific achievement.

Pharmacology, like other sciences in China, is oriented to decisions made by revolutionary committees, but the decisions are not determined solely by political considerations. Social and economic factors can be significant motivating forces, as evidenced by the large-scale preventive medicine program instituted in the early years of the regime. During this period primary emphasis was placed on eradicating parasitic diseases. As a consequence, pharmacologists had to channel their energies to studying the pharmacology of agents used in the treatment of these diseases and to screening numerous compounds for parasiticidal activity. In this program, pharmacology occupied an important (if secondary) place in epidemiologic approaches to the parasitic dieseases. During the early years, therefore, the present regime recognized clearly the immediate health needs of the people and displayed a willingness to cope with these problems. Since the Great Leap Forward, the new goal of pharmacology appears to be one of probing for something useful in ancient China's medical history, combined with an emphasis on finding drugs for the treatment of common chronic diseases.

Most of the research in pharmacology has been carried out under the leadership of Western-trained scientists. The main institutions for pharmacologic research are the Institute of Materia Medica of the Chinese Academy of Medical Sciences in Peking, the Shanghai Institute of Materia Medica, and the Department of Pharmacology of Chung Shan Medical College in Canton, all three of which were visited by our delegation. We saw little evidence of basic pharmacologic research in these laboratories, although the personnel include some excellent investigators. In the main, the research consists either of screening drugs of plant and animal origin for pharmacologic activity or determining the pharmacologic profile of some isolated active principles. The work is directed primarily toward developing drugs for the treatment of bronchitis, hypertension, and cancer. Almost all of the basic research described to us and, indeed, much of the investigation on characterization of drug principles appears to have been carried out before the Cultural Revolution. We surmised that research has progressed at a snail's pace, with little pharmacologic progress, since 1958. Supporting this view is the fact that little significant work has been published in the last ten years.

No important Chinese school appears to have developed that might influence future work in specialized areas of pharmacology, such as the stimulus given the world by the neurotransmitter work in Europe or by biochemical pharmacology in the United States in the areas of drug biotransformation, enzymology, and renal excretion. This is perhaps too much to ask of a country in such a short time, particularly since the early emphasis was on catching up and since, by political decree, work had to be done in areas of preventive medicine. (The situation is not dissimilar to the Russian scene, which has also not created an exciting school of pharmacology.) With the mass program in effect to study the flora and fauna of China, some important fundamental discoveries may now arise as a by-product, however, provided that the pharmacologists are not too preoccupied with screening and evaluating plant and animal extracts to have any time for more basic investigative pursuits.

There is as yet little application in China of modern principles of clinical pharmacology. This is certainly due in part to the fact that evaluation of drug efficacy in the clinic at a sophisticated scientific level is of relatively recent origin. In the United States, many drug-testing procedures on patients have now been standardized by clinical pharmacologists, using double-blind techniques, placebos, comparison of a new drug with a known reference standard, and statistical analysis of data. Such investigations (and investigators) are virtually unknown in China, and the published papers reflect this deficiency. (Chinese clinicians are aware of the double-blind technique but maintain that every patient should be treated and, therefore, that placebo medication is taboo.)

This rather unsophisticated approach to clinical trials is not employed in all areas, however. For example, some of the clinical studies involving the treatment of parasitic infections were more meaningful. These studies were performed mostly when the emphasis was on the eradication of parasitic diseases and before the Great Leap Forward in 1958, when the policy on traditional medicine assumed ascendancy.

Of the parasitic diseases studied, schistosomiasis was deemed to be of greatest importance, and the pharmacologic literature reflects this emphasis. An extensive screening program was carried out to discover new and effective agents against schistosomiais. Some antimonial compounds were synthesized that appear to have some potential. These include antimony ammonium gluconate, antimony sodium dimercaptosuccinate (Sb-58), and thiouracil-antimony-1. Medicinal plants reported to possess activity were Cucurbita pepo (pumpkin seed), Hemerocallis thunbergii, Lobelia radicans, Euphorbia pekinensis, and Veratrum nigrum.

The achievements with respect to schistosomiasis, malaria, kala-azar, filariasis, and ancylostomiasis are impressive. The attack on these diseases appears to have been systematic, concerted, and thorough, although the contributions of pharmacology to this success were secondary to the mass preventive health measures.

During our trip, we had opportunity to see a number of procedures in experimental pharmacology currently being employed at one or another of the institutes on our itinerary.

In the cardiovascular area, standard measurements of coronary and muscle blood flow are performed in dogs. Radioactive rubidium uptake is measured in mouse heart as an index of cardiac blood flow. Thirty seconds after a single intravenous dose of ^{86}Rb, the heart is removed and the radioactivity measured. This method was being used to assess beta-adrenergic drugs and blockers; nitroglycerin produced a prominent effect. Another technique for assessing potentially useful coronary durgs is the antagonism of pitocin-induced electrocardiographic abnormalities in rats. Rabbits are the experimental animals used for study of the ability of drugs to inhibit aortic plaque formation after the feeding of an atherogenic diet.

In cancer chemotherapy, the experimental tumors used include a number that are classical in Western laboratories as well as a few indigenous varieties. (The Chinese do not use some strains considered very useful in the United States such as the L1210 leukemia.) For screening anticancer antibiotics, they employ a series of in vitro assays, including phage and methylene blue uptake by cancer cells. Inhibitory effects on spermatogonia and on rate of thymidine incorporation into nucleotides are also employed.

Because of the widespread occurrence of bronchitis in China, it is natural that laboratories should be devoting part of their efforts to developing new drugs as expectorants or cough suppressants. We saw several antitussive screens employing either ammonia or sulfur dioxide gas to induce cough in mice. Unfortunately, the tussive dose seems close to the lethal dose. Anesthetized rats are also used to study the effects of drugs on tracheal secretions, either by simply weighing capillary tubes inserted into the trachea, or measuring the amount of phenol red entering the tracheal secretions after intraperitoneal injections.

A model for emphysema is the induction of pulmonary damage by papain in rats. Rats are also exposed to cold to induce changes in the bronchiolar mucous membrane and glands, and the effect of drugs on these pathological changes is measured.

Several anti-inflammatory and antibacterial techniques in rabbits were in use at Nan K'ai Hospital in the study of acupuncture. These included phagocytosis of staphylococci, the production of experimental appendiceal gangrene (so as to allow study of the speed with which peritoneal exudate is absorbed), cotton granuloma induction, the leukocyte response to S. typhosa endotoxin, and toxoid-induced pyresis.

As "antihepatitis" screens, two procedures were described to us. One is the standard protection against carbon tetrachloride-induced liver necrosis and death, and the second is the measurement of bile flow in the anesthetized rat via a cannula implanted in the common bile duct.

Finally, some traditional analgesic screens are in use, such as the mouse hot plate and the rabbit nose twitch (after electrical stimulation of tooth pulp) techniques and classical in vitro muscle strip methods for assaying cholinergic agonists and antagonists.

As in the West, pharmacologic screening in China has both its rational and irrational elements. The Chinese are not unique in using experimental procedures that seem a far cry from the human condition of interest, but one wonders how useful some of their screening approaches will prove to be empirically, either in explaining or documenting suspected clinical activity of herbal medicines.

LABORATORY RESEARCHES EMANATING FROM HERBAL MEDICINE

With the impetus provided both by Chairman Mao's enthusiasm for traditional medicine and by the apparent beneficial effects obtained from the use of natural products, it is not surprising that there should be laboratory follow-up and a search for active principles. Yet one must still ask why, if there is so little doubt in the minds of the Chinese about the safety and efficacy of these herbal drugs, should anyone feel a need for expensive and lengthy laboratory pursuits?

The answer certainly does not lie in a Chinese-perceived need to convince anyone in the West. Rather, we were told, it is important to know how the drugs act (and perhaps how to use them better); it is necessary to produce more convenient forms of dispensing the herbal drugs (e.g., tablets, capsules, ampuls), thus eliminating the fuss and bother of decoctions; and finally, since some of the traditional drug sources were in short supply, the definition of active principles may ensure more abundant supplies through the efforts of the chemists.

In our travels, we saw not only herbal drugs studied in pharmacology laboratories (using the variety of animal analogues of human physiologic or pathologic processes described in the preceding section) but also some molecular modification of chemicals originally obtained from natural sources.

The Institute of Chinese Materia Medica of the Academy of Traditional Chinese Medicine was founded in 1955 as a part of the general re-emphasis of traditional Chinese medicine and pharmacology, which followed the exhortations of Chairman Mao. The buildings and laboratories reflected good maintenance and support. The director of the institute read a long and at times strongly worded introduction, which included a discussion of recent political trends. (He later requested that no photographs be taken; this proved to be the only such request during our month-long visit, except for similar admonitions at airports or on planes and at one museum.)

The staff scientists here, and in most other institutions we were to visit, were enthusiastic and unquestionably dedicated to the objective of raising the level of traditional Chinese medicine and pharmacology. There are four research areas at the Institute: (1) identification of herbs, (2) drug forms and processing, (3) chemistry, and (4) pharmacology. The first area was perhaps the most impressive; the plant and animal specimens were well prepared and the pharmacognosists knowledgeable. The pharmaceutical preparations department displayed attractively packaged products in various dosage forms.

The drug-processing laboratory was engaged in developmental research to improve an herbal extract of a five-plant mixture used for diphtheria. The preparation, which had been used in folk medicine, was a decoction. The pharmaceutical chemists told us that they had made a superior product by percolation with 45 percent alcohol, followed by evaporation to dryness and trituration of the residue with water. Another drug-processing laboratory was concerned with the effects of various treatments of the herbs (such as "carbonization" and rate of drying) upon the pharmacological activity of the extracts.

The organic chemistry laboratory was involved in a study of the active principles of an *Artemisia* species used traditionally for treating jaundice. The group reported that they had isolated several compounds, two of which showed choleretic activity - caffeic acid and *p*-hydroxyacetophenone. It was not clear whether these compounds had received significant clinical evaluation. There were two identical distillation setups used for removal of solvents. Aside from that, there were two desiccators, some plates for thin-layer chromatography, some simple balances, and about a dozen bottles of solvent lined up on the reagent shelf. Otherwise, all benches were clear. The doors of all the other laboratories were closed. The nature of the equipment in the laboratory, the experiments in progress, and the level of scientific expertise of the staff raised questions about their ability to pursue effectively the characterization of *new* active principles, a difficult challenge not met adequately in many laboratories in any country. The fourth section was concerned with developing animal assays for testing the activity of herbs but for lack of time was not visited.

The Institute of Materia Medica in Peking is under the auspices of the Chinese Academy of Medical Sciences. The institute was established in 1958, during the year of the Great Leap Forward, and has a technical staff of about 300. Its purpose is to carry out research on new drugs for common diseases, to isolate active principles of known medicinal plants, and to systematize traditional medicinal materials available in China. At present, work is being done on the prevention and treatment of the common cold and bronchitis, tumors, and cardiovascular diseases and on the development of chemical contraceptives. The institute is divided into seven departments: synthetic organic chemistry, phytochemistry, pharmacognosy, analytical chemistry, pharmacology, antibiotics, and cultivation of medicinal plants (for which there is a separate experimental station 30 kilometers from Peking).

In the phytochemistry department we heard a talk on *Pueraria lobata*, which is being used clinically for treatment of hypertension, stiff neck, and headache. It also is said to be effective in the treatment of "sudden deafness" in industrial workers exposed to loud noises. *Pueraria lobata* was used in traditional medicine for the relief of stiff neck. Four related isoflavones of type I were isolated from this plant.

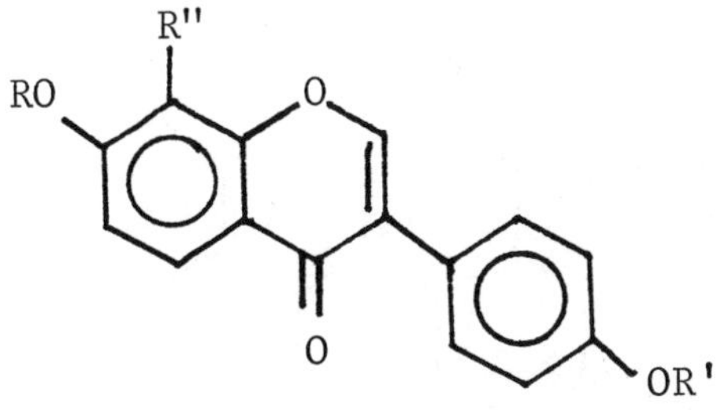

I

a, R = R' = H
b, R = glucose
c, R = R' = glucose
d, R'' = glucose

Only the diglycoside Ic was previously unknown. Three of the four isoflavones are reported to exhibit activity against sudden deafness.

From the seeds of Thevetia peruviana Merr. six different cardenolide glycosides of type II were obtained.

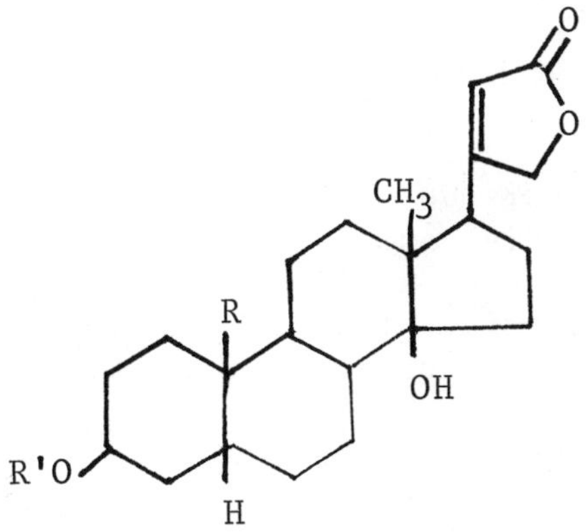

II

(R can be aldehyde, methyl, hydroxymethyl or carboxylic acid groups, and R' is some sugar moiety.) Out of this group of cardioglycosides, only perusitin (R = COOH, R' = thevetose) was a previously unknown compound. The most abundant glycosides were peruvoside, nerifolin, and acetylnerifolin. The mixture of the three is being studied clinically. Both oral and injectable preparations seem effective. There are allegedly fewer side effects with this mixture than with digitoxin.

The active component bergenin (III), an isocoumarin, was isolated in 0.2 percent yield from Ardisia japonica, which has been used for chronic bronchitis in Chinese traditional medicine. The structure of III was established by chemical and spectral data, and a synthesis was achieved, starting with glucose and gallic acid. Bergenin was known in the literature, having been isolated years ago from Bergenia crassifolia. It is about one fourth as effective as codeine in antitussive activity, but it said not to depress the respiratory center.

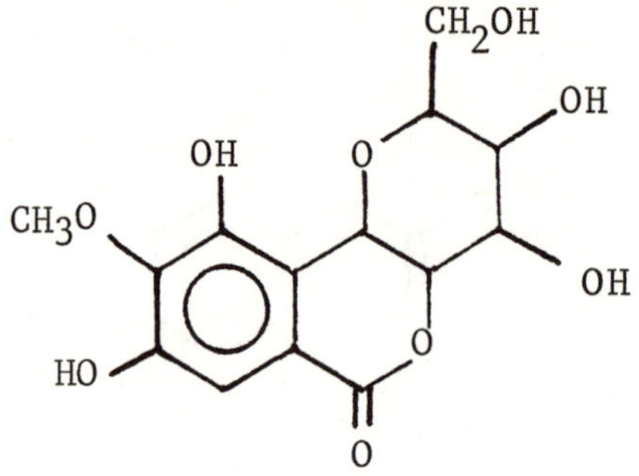

III

Securinine (IV) was isolated from the plant Securinega suffruticosa. The structure of IV has been known in the Western literature since 1962.

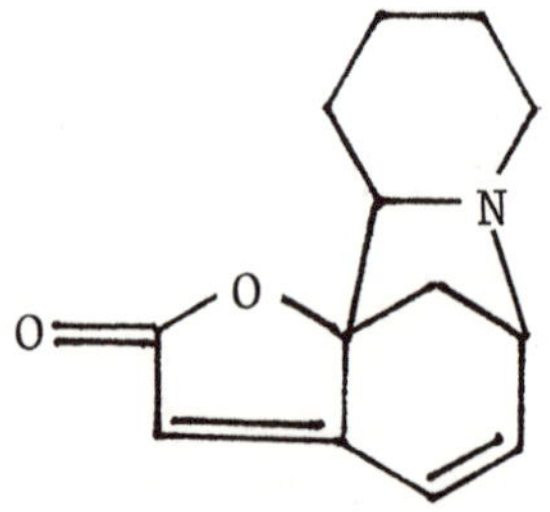

IV

This alkaloid is a known central nervous system stimulant and is currently being tested as a treatment for facial and limb paralysis. It is said to be effective in 80-95 percent of the cases studied. It also may be effective in the treatment of multiple sclerosis. Interestingly, securinine is injected at acupuncture sites, but acupuncture itself is not used unless the alkaloid proves ineffective.

Because of the illness of Huang Liang (Ph.D., Cornell University; postdoctoral experience at Bryn Mawr College, Wayne State University and Iowa State University), no presentation by the synthetic chemistry department was scheduled for our visit. However, after much insistence, Liang Hsiao-t'ien (Ph.D., University of Washington; postdoctoral training at Harvard University) showed a few of us a laboratory where two young chemists were synthesizing some aliphatic α-keto-aldehydes. The bis-thiosemicarbazones were to be prepared for testing of their antitumor activities. The laboratory equipment looked very much like one of the 1950's, except for the extensive use of thin-layer chromatography. (Perhaps this reflects the fact that the leading Chinese chemists mostly returned to China from their overseas training and research in the 1950's. Although there is good access to the current Western chemical literature, there has not been as good access to modern laboratory equipment.)

In the analytical department, we saw two ultraviolet-optical rotary dispersion spectrophotometers (JASCO), an air-conditioned room that contained a 60-MHz nuclear magnetic resonance (NMR) spectrometer (JEOL) and, in a separate room, a mass spectrometer (JEOL). There was also a preparative gas chromatograph made in Shanghai. Aside from the NMR instrument, which had a sample spinning, none of the other machines seemed to be in use the afternoon of our visit.

In another section of the natural products laboratory we were told that the institute is preparing ergot alkaloids for clinical use by fermentation. Before settling on the final wheat species presently employed, they explored some 800 other plant substrates for the fungus. Fermentation production is carried out on at least a 200 liter scale. In general, it would seem that most of the experimental results we were shown were probably well in hand prior to 1965.

After lunch we were taken to the pharmacology floor. Monocrotaline has been isolated from *Crotalaria sessiflora*, a plant used in folk medicine for skin cancer. This *Senecio* alkaloid is active in the Walker 256 screening system, but liver toxicity is too high for use in man; similar results have been obtained in our National Cancer Institute's programs. Later in the afternoon we learned that the synthetic organic group, directed by Huang Liang, has been making derivatives of monocrotaline, but so far, none, including the *N*-oxide, has proved more suitable than the present compound. (The discovery of monocrotaline as an alkaloid effective in inhibiting the Walker 256 carcinosarcoma in the rat was first described by Morris Kupchan's laboratory in the United States in a report published in 1964. Subsequent preclinical toxicological studies in the National Cancer Institute's program revealed serious hepatoxicity, and the alkaloid was deemed unsuitable for clinical trials.) Some screening is done in this institute using Yoshida sarcoma, sarcoma SK, sarcoma 37, and leukemia L615. However, there is no systematic screening of plants for anticancer activity. The cancer laboratory (which seemed to be only a small effort) was also pursuing the pharmacology of *N*-formyl-DL-sarcolysine, which is being used clinically (with good results) for seminoma. Another synthetic drug under investigation is kethoxal bis-thiosemicarbazone, which is being employed for cancer of the bladder. Also mentioned was the ethyl ester of *N*-nitrosarcosin.

During the brief visit to the synthetic organic chemistry laboratory with Liang Hsiao-t'ien, we were told of continuing attempts to modify the aforenamed classes of compounds to find relatives with better therapeutic indices. The approaches outlined appeared to follow well-trodden (and hitherto unrewarding) routes, and the equipment in the laboratories appeared to be of 1950-1955 level.

Last on the schedule was the taxonomic section. Here we met a group under the direction of Hsiao P'ei-ken (about 30-35 years of age and educated entirely in China), an outstanding botanist and chemotaxonomist. His group is set up for botanic identification and art reproduction. The herbarium collection amounts to 50,000 plant specimens from all over the world and is probably representative of most of the 35,000 species indigenous to China. The collection contains most, if not all, of the 5,000 known medicinal plants in China. The department is preparing a new handbook of medicinal herbs and is making excellent paintings to help in characterization.

Later in our visit, Professor Kao I-sheng (Ph.D., Oxford; trained with Sir Robert Robinson) gave us a general introduction to the work of the Shanghai Institute of Materia Medica. Since the Cultural Revolution, it has been under the direction of the Municipal Revolutionary Committee of Shanghai. There are approximately 470 staff members, of whom 300 are scientists. It is divided into departments of synthetic drugs, microchemistry, pharmacology, analytical chemistry, antibiotics, and auxiliary sections. The main concern of this institute is to study new drugs and to carry out research on antitumor agents and on treatment of diseases of the nervous system, chronic bronchitis, hepatitis, cardiovascular diseases, and contraceptives. The chemistry departments are concerned with the synthesis and isolation of biologically active compounds. For known drugs, already discovered in the West, the work is primarily on the development of good synthetic routes and the modification of isolation procedures applicable to sources native to China. There is no "theoretical" research, and all work must have a connection with medical practice. Most of the earlier work from this laboratory has been published. We were shown their current research efforts.

For this purpose, we were divided into two groups, but each group saw the same laboratories and personnel (contrary to our expectations), except in a different sequence. In the chemistry department, we heard a talk on synthetic anticancer drugs. Since 1958, this institute has prepared 2,000 compounds for screening. Among these are the following:

1. Alkylating agents of the sarcolysin type V, where R, R', and R" were varied. The best anticancer agent in this group is mecaphane, Va, where

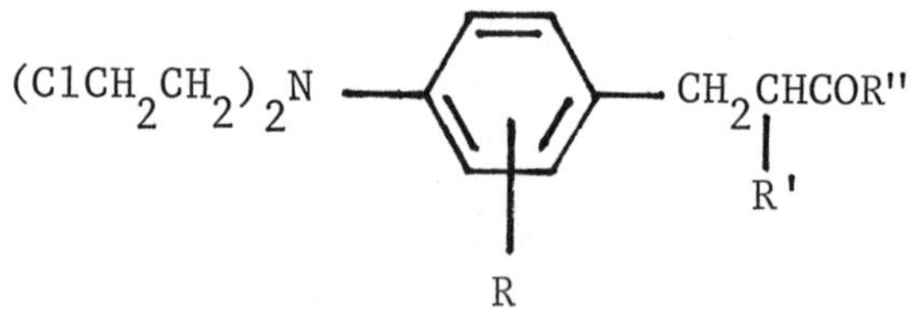

Va

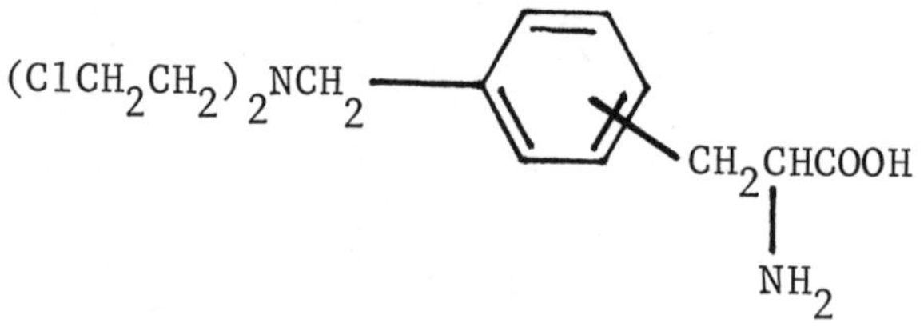

Vb

R = OCH_3, R' = NH_2 and R'' = OH. The D and L forms of this amino acid were equally effective. Other structural modifications of type Vb (a homologue of sarcolysin), including the <u>ortho</u>, <u>meta</u>, and <u>para</u> isomers, were prepared. These compounds have high toxicity but are still under clinical testing. Nitrocaphane (AT1258) is currently being tested as a treatment for cancer of the nasopharynx.

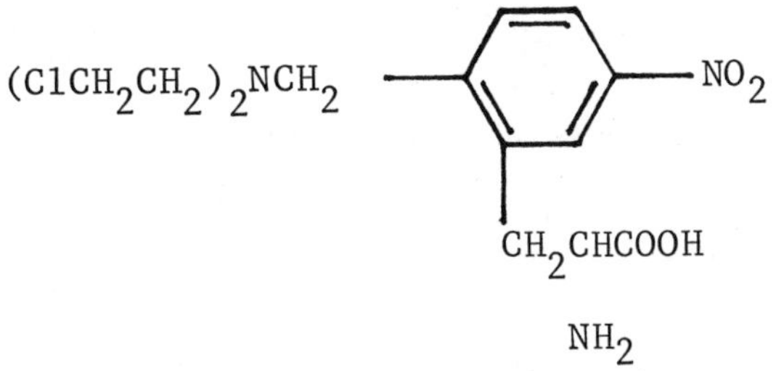

AT1258

Another nitrogen mustard, VI, is used as an analgesic.

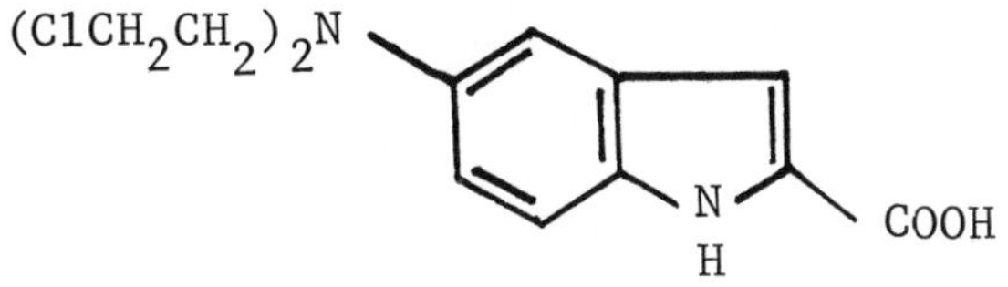

VI

2. Antimetabolites in the field of purines and pyrimidines. A series of derivatives of 6-mercaptopurines of the type VII were synthesized.

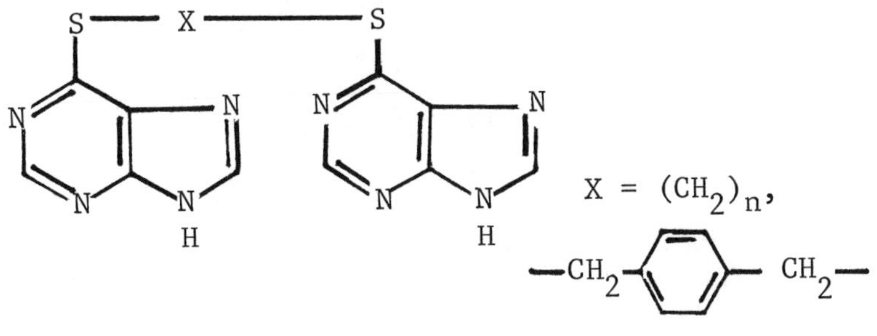

VII

The more soluble sodium Bunte salt of 6-mercaptopurine (AT1438) was being tested for treatment of leukemia.

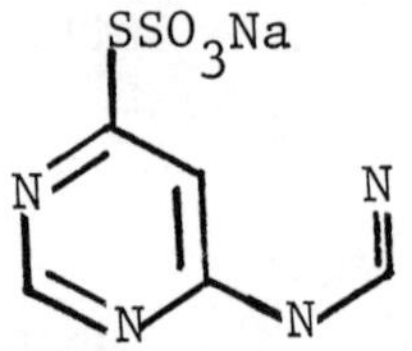

AT1438

3. Some antimonial chelates. These were first prepared for antischistosomiasis studies. It was found that VIII chelates antimony most strongly and IX chelates it least effectively.

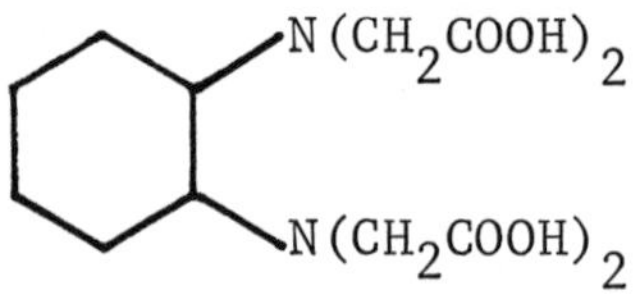

VIII

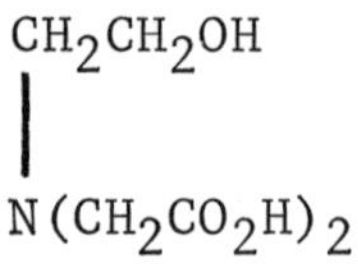

IX

The medium strength chelates (i.e. Sb71) have the best antitumor activity.

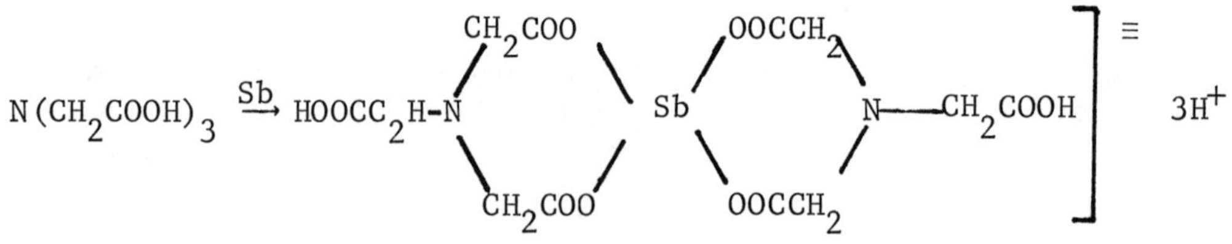

Sb71

Sb71 is being tested for tumors of soft tissue (e.g., neck). It seems to be of relatively low toxicity.

4. Other anticancer agents synthesized by this group include type X and AT236.

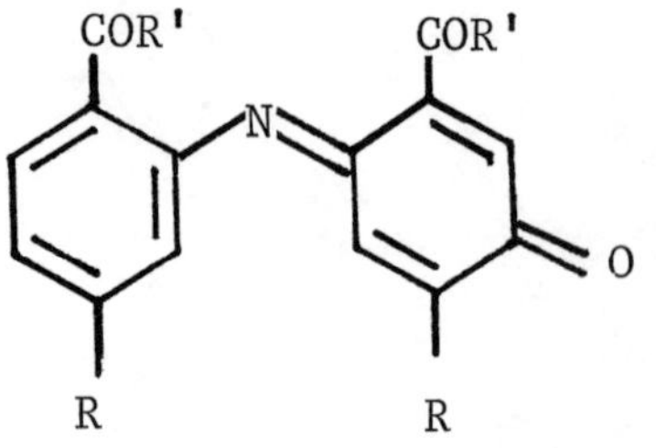

X

R' = OCH_3, OC_2H_5, $OCH(CH_3)_2$ = $OCH_2C_6H_5$

R = ?

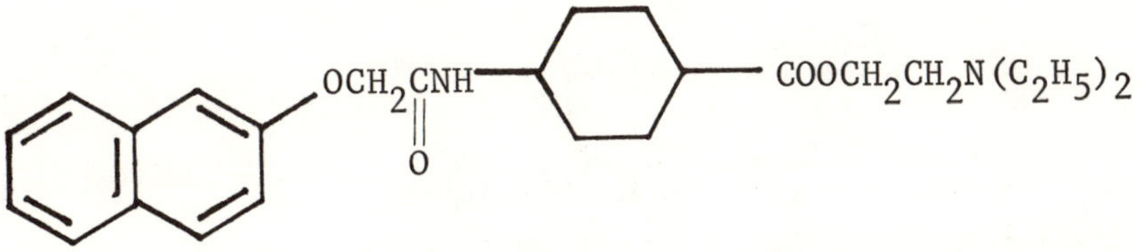

AT236

The synthetic effort appears to have followed well-known pathways also exploited elsewhere, and the results were equally unexciting. Natural products used in cancer chemotherapy appeared to be limited to those previously reported in the West and now produced from Chinese sources: e.g. mitomycin, actinomycin D, vincristine, vinblastine, and camptothecin.

Camptotheca acuminata Decsne is a Chinese tree from which the experimental tumor-inhibiting alkaloid camptothecin was isolated in the United States. We were told that scientists at the institute have discovered that the seeds (rather than the wood) constitute the best source of camptothecin and that good clinical results have been obtained in the treatment of gastrointestinal tumors. The results appear to differ from the experience of U.S. investigators, who showed the compound to be ineffective in doses up to those causing significant toxicity.

For the treatment of chronic bronchitis, an active principle rorifone (XI) was extracted from the plant *Rorippa montana*, one of the Cruciferae.

$$CH_3SO_2(CH_2)_9CN$$

XI

The previously unknown structure was determined largely by use of infrared and NMR spectra. It is being used clinically, taken in crystalline form at the rate of 200-300 mg/day. When large amounts of rorifone were injected into large animals, they shared the same toxic action as results from cyanide ion. This effect can be counteracted by the simultaneous administration of sodium thiosulfate. The rorifone was synthesized from castor oil via the following scheme:

$$\text{castor oil} \xrightarrow{\text{NaOH}} HO(CH_2)_9COOH \xrightarrow[\text{2) EtOH/HCl}]{\text{1) HBr}}$$

$$Br(CH_2)_9COOEt \xrightarrow{CH_3SNa} CH_3S(CH_2)_9\ COOEt \xrightarrow{H_2O_2}$$

$$CH_3\overset{\overset{O}{\|}}{\underset{\underset{O}{\|}}{S}}(CH_2)_9COOEt \xrightarrow{H_2O} CH_3SO_2(CH_2)_9COOH$$

$$\xrightarrow[\text{2) } P_2O_5]{\text{1) } NH_2\overset{\overset{}{}}{\underset{\underset{O}{\|}}{C}}NH_2} CH_3SO_2(CH_2)_9CN$$

They have also prepared various modified structures of the following type.

1. $R(CH_2)_9CN$ R = CN, OH, H, C_2H_5, OCH_3, SCH_3, COOH, C_3H_7, C_4H_9, C_6H_5 and p-ClC_6H_5.

2. $CH_3SO_2(CH_2)_nCN$ n = 1-11

3. $CH_3SO_2(CH_2)_9R$ R = SO_2CH_3, SH, Br, Cl, $CONH_2$, $NHCH_3$, CH_3, $COOC_2H_5$, $COOC_6H_{13}$, $OCOC_2H_5$, COOH, $COOC_6H_4OCH_3$.

Among all these, only the last three compounds were active against bronchitis. The activity is less than that of rorifone itself; however, these compounds are said to have a better therapeutic ratio. The acid derivative, although less active than rorifone, has a better therapeutic ratio and was being clinically tested.

In other areas of natural products, four compounds isolated from the plant *Andrographis paniculata* have shown broad-spectrum antibiotic activity. All are known in the literature, but their use against bacillary dysentery had not been described. Among these, neoandrographolide (XII) was most active. It allegedly has fewer side effects than chloramphenicol.

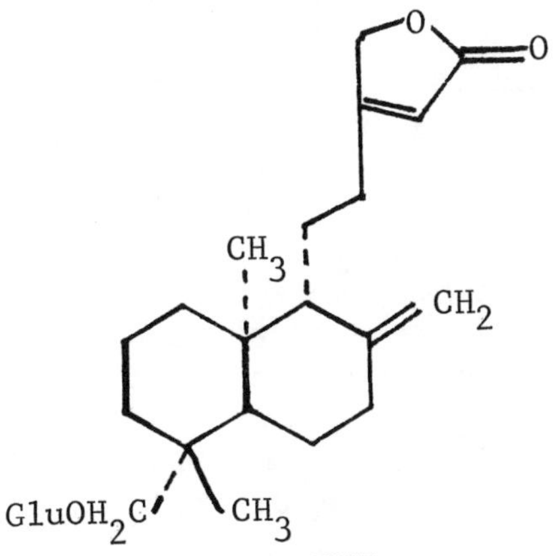

XII

d-Catechin (XIII) was isolated from Potentilla fragarioides. It is used for treatment of bleeding in gynecology.

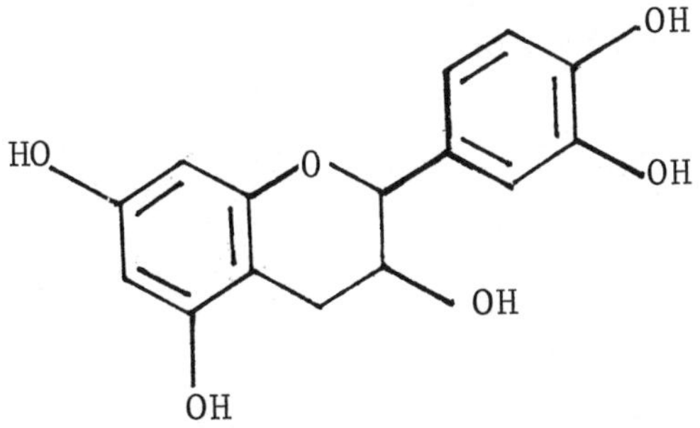

XIII

From Corydalis ambigua, known for its analgesic effect from ancient herbals, (±)-tetrahydropalmatine was isolated as the effective ingredient. The same product can be prepared by hydrogenation of palmatine, which is isolated from Fibrauria tinctoria. The alkaloid is converted to its sulfate salt for preparation of the product corylgine. From Stephania sinica, the (-)-form of tetrahydropalmatine ("rotundine") was isolated. Rotundine is a more effective analgesic than its (+)-isomer, and is available in both tablet and injectable form in 30 mg doses.

In the analytical chemistry department, we saw several automatic carbon, hydrogen and nitrogen analyzers. There were also Mettler-type balances made in Shanghai. A high-pressure liquid-chromatography (HPLC) apparatus was built in the institute as a joint project by a phytochemist, a physicist, and an electronics expert. Currently, they are building a preparative HPLC machine. We were told that they have a 100-MHz NMR spectrometer (JEOL), and are expecting to get a mass spectrometer as well.

The Institute of Organic Chemistry in Shanghai was founded in 1950 under the sponsorship of the Academia Sinica. The Director, Wang Yu, a graduate of Ching Ling University, Nanking, received his Ph.D. from the University of Munich under the late Professor H. Wieland and did postdoctoral research with Dodds in England. He told us that in 1949 there were only 20 organic chemists in the whole of China, mostly scattered among various universities in Peking and Shanghai. Four chemists were assigned to start this institute. In 24 years, it has grown to a total staff of 1,100, of whom between 600 and 700 are chemists.

In the early years, the research of this institute was devoted to helping the economic reconstruction of China. Work was concentrated in the fields of antibiotics and polymers. A department to study medicinal chemistry related to Chinese herbs was established, and in 1955 this department split off to become the Institute of Materia Medica. In 1958, during the period of the Great Leap Forward, natural-product chemistry was expanded, and research in the areas of fluorocarbons and organometallic compounds was initiated.

Today, the institute is divided into the following departments: natural products, chemistry of extractives (*t*-amine types and organic phosphates for water purification), chemistry of metallo-organic compounds, biochemistry, analytical chemistry, and physical chemistry. The department of natural products is carrying out work on steroids, polypeptides and proteins, nucleic acids, and the microbial oxidation of petroleum.

It seems that about one third of the institute's technical staff is concerned with various aspects of natural-products chemistry. Of these, 30 chemists have been assigned to nucleotide chemistry, 17 to polypeptide chemistry, and others seemed concerned with steroid development (oral contraceptives), synthesis of protein sources, and fluorine polymer chemistry (for example, polytetrafluoroethylene). The senior staff are quite capable of directing work in these areas.

Among the institute's senior members (who all seem to be in their 50's) is Liu Chu-chin, who has directed natural products work but is now working on liquid crystals. He did postdoctoral work with Professor V. Boekelheide at the University of Rochester. The steroid group is headed by Chou Wei-shan, who was a member of the Insect Hormone Delegation to the United States in 1973. The organofluorine group is headed by a Harvard trained organic chemist, Huang Wei-yuan.

Of the perhaps 120 laboratories in the main building of this large institute that, with manufacturing units, seemed to encompass two city blocks, we were shown four laboratories. The first was concerned with converting the C_{12}-C_{18} paraffin fractions (0.5 percent aromatic compounds) from the Chinese petroleum field (discovered in 1960) to a source of animal protein using the yeast *Candida lipolytica*. The conversion of such paraffin oil to yeast protein amounts to 70-80 percent. Gas oil (diesel) yields a toxic protein, but the fraction extracted with alcohol is suitable for feeding animals. At present the institute is interested in circumventing the aromatic compounds, which probably produce some serious toxicologic problems, for example, of the carcinogenic type. A manuscript based on this problem has recently been prepared.

Next, we heard a brief talk on the structural determination of spieimine (XV), a steroidal alkaloid isolated from the plant *Fritillaria pallidiflora*.

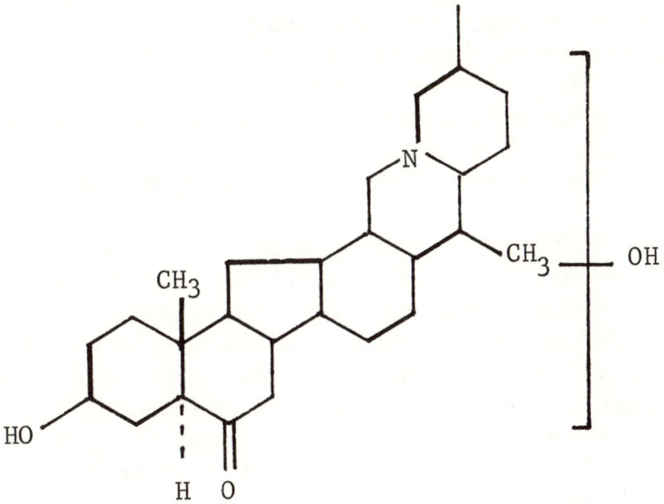

XV

The work was carried out mostly by classical methods of degradation. At the time this work was done, the group had no NMR spectrometer, and so it was only possible to propose this partial structure. The final placement of the second hydroxyl group at C_{22} was reported by the Russians.

There was also a talk on the synthesis of ($\pm$) menthol from (+) piperitone. It was obvious these two pieces of research had been accomplished before the Cultural Revolution.

Liu Chu-chin also described some of his earlier structure work with the Veratrum alkaloids. All of the studies viewed that afternoon were completed prior to 1965. In Chou Wei-shan's steroid laboratory we heard a brief description of their conversion of diosgenin and 3α,7α-cholic acid (hydrodeoxycholic acid) to cortisol, prednisone, dexamethasone, triamcinolone, 16-methylene-prednisone acetate, 6-methyl-cortisol acetate, megesterol acetate, mestranol, and norethisterone. Obviously, they have been assigned the task of making these important drugs available for Chinese medical use.

In a different laboratory, we heard a talk on the group's earlier work on the structure of streptomycin. The structure was proposed originally by Wolfrom to have a β-linkage between streptidine and the disaccharide streptobiosamine. The Chinese scientists found it to be an α-linkage by molecular rotation calculations. Later, this proposal was confirmed by independent groups at the University of Illinois (by means of NMR studies) and at Imperial College, London (by use of x-ray crystallography).

A young chemist, Dr. Hsu, told us of the isolation of esculetin (6,7-dihydroxycoumarin) and esculin (7-Hydroxycoumarin-6-O-B-D-glucoside) from Fraxinus rhynchophylla (ash bark). These compounds were said to be effective in the treatment of bacillary dysentery. Esculetin is now being synthesized on an industrial scale. It is less effective than chloramphenicol, but the toxicity is also lower.

Dr. Hsu further told us about the insulin synthesis accomplished in this laboratory. This project was a joint effort with the Shanghai Institute of Biochemistry and Peking University. The work carried out under the direction of Dr. Hsu was concerned with the preparation of the A-chain. It was completed in September 1965. They are now working on the modification of the insulin structure, and have found that the B-chain can be shortened by at least eight amino acid units without loss of activity.

The polypeptide group consists of 13 chemists. The institute established a group of 30 chemists to work on nucleic acids. Unfortunately, we did not have a chance to visit with them. At the very end of our visit, we asked about the available instrumentation and were told that there was a Japanese-made nuclear magnetic resonance instrument and a British mass spectrometer. Although this world-renowned group of organic chemists was diverted in 1965 to development work, some of the visiting group had the impression that they were working on large molecules of biological importance.

At the Peking Municipal Hospital of Chinese Traditional Medicine, our visit included a stop in a laboratory engaged in the isolation of active principles of *Physalis alkekengi* (syn. *P. franchetii*), which is used for tonsilitis. The chemists showed enthusiasm and capacity for reisolation of known constituents, although we could not be sure that their training was up to the far more demanding task of isolating new and active compounds.

At the Nanking College of Pharmacy, the Professor of Organic Chemistry, Peng Shu-hsun, had spent a postdoctoral year with Professor R.C. Elderfield at Columbia University in 1951 - 1952. He described ... research projects in phytochemistry, which were concerned with developmental problems, brought to the college by students who encountered them during their field experience. One project sought improved procedures for isolating know "anti-inflammatory" andrographolides from *Andrographis paniculata* (see discussion of Institute of Materia Medica, Shanghai, p.35). Another study involved the process for isolating pseudolycorine, a quanternary alkaloid from *Lycoris radiata*, of interest as a potential antiemetic and antitussive drug. The presently available process utilizes expensive reineckate salts for the isolation, and a cheaper process is being sought. The mother liquors remaining after isolation of camptothecin from *Camptotheca acuminata* are under study for isolation of campanion alkaloids, such as hydroxycamptothecin. There was some ambiguity as to how far the biological studies of hydroxycamptothecin have progressed.

At Peking University we visited the Department of Organic Chemistry and Biochemistry. The biology laboratories appeared to have somewhat limited equipment. We were shown a 1955-vintage ultraviolet spectrophotometer, a little-used apparatus for paper electrophoresis, and a vapor-phase chromatograph used in teaching exercises (to distinguish between saturated and unsaturated fats). A laboratory for research on active principles was engaged in studies on species of *Trollius* and *Humulus*. The *Trollius* species had yielded a compound with "anti-infective" and "anti-inflammatory" properties, and the compound had been partially characterized as a flavonoid. The *Humulus* species (hops) were being studied as sources for new antitubercular drugs. Humulone and lupulone, two well-known hops constitutents, have been said to have antitubercular properties, and the researchers proposed to look for more active companion principles. A question as to how the activity would be monitored brought a response that indicated that this had not yet been decided, because "the work was just starting."

Finally, we also saw some research being done on a drug from the plant Ilex pubescens. The plant is a shrub or small tree belonging to the Aquifolicaceae family. An extract of the root is being studied in the treatment of coronary heart disease. At the Department of Pharmacology of Chung Shan Medical College, Professor Wu Hsiu-jung and her aides demonstrated the drug's effect in an open-chest heart-lung preparation of a dog. The drug doubled the coronary flow while decreasing blood pressure by about 50 percent some 30 minutes after intravenous injection, with a duration in excess of 3 hours. Professor Wu stated that the drug has a direct inotropic effect and also lowers the oxygen consumption of cardiac tissue. The drug has been tried in the clinic at Chung Shan Hospital in over 100 cases, including 10 patients with myocardial infarction.[1] The report claims that on oral or intramuscular administration, improvement was noted in 97 percent of the cases. Before treatment the patients had severe chest pains, which largely or completely disappeared after therapy. Headaches, dizziness, and numbness also disappeared. In a majority of the subjects who had hypertension, blood pressure returned to normal.

Although members of the delegation did not have an opportunity to see purified principles developed from Chinese traditional herbs being used in patients, these are summarized below. In most cases compounds indicated were not original discoveries of the Chinese; however, they were isolated from Chinese plants, presumably on the basis of the use of the plants in decoction form for the same purposes as the purified principle.

Purified Principle	Source	Use
(±)-Tetrahydropalmatine	Corydalis ambigua	Sedative, tranquilizer, analgesic
(-)-Tetrahydropalmatine (syn. rotundine)	Stephania sinica	Same as above
Rorifone	Rorippa montana	Antitussive
(+)-Tetrandrine	Stephania tetrandra	Antihypertensive
Berberine	Berberis spp.	Antidiarrheal, antibacterial
Neoandrographolide	Andrographis paniculata	Antibacterial
Esculetin	Fraxinus rhynchophylla	Antidysentery
6-Hydroxyatropine	Scopolia lurida	For symptoms of meningitis

Since these drugs are either accepted clinically in China at the present time or are in various stages of clinical investigation, their clinical utility may deserve evaluation in the West.

In concluding this section, it seems appropriate to comment upon the general purpose of the visit of our delegation, namely, to discuss research on natural products for therapeutic use, identification of medically effective elements, and development of synthetic drugs with these elements. Our discussions revealed a national dedication to follow Chairman Mao's exhortations to study China's herbal medicines. Medical schools, hospitals, and institutes devoted to traditional medicines are expanding, and ever-increasing support appears to be channeled in their direction. Useful new medicaments, constituted of extracts made from plant mixtures, may emerge, but a significant number of new and useful active principles or synthetic drugs based on plant principles will probably not be forthcoming in the immediate future. Effective progress in these areas will require a substantially increased investment in the advanced training of chemists and biologists for the highly demanding research required. Extensive new instrumentation for chemical and biological research will also be needed. One can only hope that the time is not too distant when higher priorities for filling these needs will expedite the rate at which China's biomedical scientists may explore effectively their "treasure-house" - the active principles of traditional medicinal plants. At present, Chinese achievements in the field of natural products chemistry are minimal, and although our delegation could not identify any unequivocally useful new medicines because of the inability to observe controlled clinical studies, several plants discussed in this report appear to merit further study on potential sources of biologically interesting compounds.

MEDICINAL PLANT GARDENS IN CHINA

Although we had requested an opportunity to see the large-scale cultivation and harvesting of medicinal plants, this never came to pass. We had read in a Chinese periodical, China Reconstructs that "in the past, most herbs grew wild. Many took years to mature. Some grew only in one part of the country. Today herbs are grown on state farms as well as in communes and brigade health stations all over China." What we did see were plant gardens, even when they were described to us as "plantations." None of them were in fact places where herbs were grown for supplying the needs of Chinese patients. We left wondering whether the large plantations existed and were simply too distant from the large cities we visited, or whether large-scale production is still mostly a goal for the future. In fairness, it must be stated that our visit was limited to cities, and that extensive side trips would not have been possible, given our schedule.

South China is said to be a leading medicinal plant-producing region. In the province of Kwangsi it is claimed that more that 200 types are cultivated, 40 of them introduced from other parts of the country and 150 cultivated from local wild plants. The people have been encouraged to exploit the mountainous areas, which are most suitable for cultivating these plants. Yunnan, Kweichow, and Szechwan are other provinces which supply large quantities of medicinal herbs. In the northeast province of Kirin, deer are bred for their antlers, such antlers being much prized as tonics in traditional Chinese medicine.

Experimental Plantation of the Institute of Materia Medica, Peking

This facility is located on the outskirts of Peking and was the most impressive of its kind that we observed during our trip. About 1,500 species are under cultivation in an area of about 64 acres. The station is larger and more extensive than any such facility in the United States. Its functions were stated to be as follows:

a. To be a teaching facility for barefoot doctors who come here to learn how to identify the most important medicinal plants. We were told that about 10,000 barefoot doctors are trained here each year.

b. To gain experience in the cultivation of medicinal herbs.

c. To cultivate seedlings.

d. To gather information on Chinese medicinal herbs and to make positive identifications of each species when the plants were known previously only under the vernacular name.

e. To supply research laboratories with sufficient authenticated plant material for biological evaluations or phytochemical studies.

f. To maintain adequate seed supplies (germ plasm) of as many medicinal plants as possible.

The experimental station was organized in rectangular plots about 10 ft. x 40 ft., with about 10 species growing in each plot. The number of plants of each species varied, depending on the size of the individual plants, but usually several hundred could be expected. Each species was identified with an appropriate sign giving the Latin binomial (only a very few spelling errors were encountered), as well as the use of the plant written in Chinese characters. It appeared that the taxonomic nomenclature was very up-to-date, indicating a high degree of expertise among the botanists and chemotaxonomists. Most of the plants observed were growing robustly, with only a few in bad condition (this is to be expected, since all plants do not reach maturity at the same time).

A section of the experimental station contained plants in pots under a shade cover; these were plants that would suffer adversely when exposed to continuous sunlight. A separate, rather extensive section, was devoted to the cultivation of ginseng (*Panax ginseng*), also under a shade cover.

Although it was impossible to document all of the uses of the plants under cultivation, the following plants and their uses in Chinese medicine were noted:

Plant Name	Family	Use	Comments
Dianthus chinensis	Caryophyllaceae	Diaphoretic	
Macleaya cordata	Papaveraceae	Analgesic	
Phytolacca americana	Phytolaccaceae	Diuretic, emetic	
Zea mays	Gramineae	Diuretic	Used widely as a folkloric diuretic in many countries.
Morus alba	Moraceae	Sedative	

Prunus persica	Rosaceae	Antitussive	Cyanogenic compound in the seeds said to be antitussive.
Thalictrum sp.	Ranunculaceae	Antibacterial	Extracts of many _Thalictrum_ species have shown antibacterial activity.
Eucommia ulmoides	Eucommiaceae	Treatment of hypertension, neck pain	
Celastrus orbicularis	Celastraceae	Antirheumatic	
Sophora flavescens	Leguminosae	Anthelmintic, diuretic	
Sanguisorba officinalis	Rosaceae	Antidiuretic, antidiarrheal	
Aconitum sp.	Ranunculaceae	Analgesic (poisonous)	
Peucedanum decursivum	Umbelliferae	Antitussive	
Chelidonium majus	Papaveraceae	Analgesic	
Penstemon barbatus	Scrophulariaceae	Dermatitis	
Gynura crepidioides	Compositae	Diuretic, spleen disorders	
Achillea millefolium	Compositae	Snakebite	
Silybum marianum	Compositae	Liver disorders	A flavonoid, silymarin, is currently on the market in West Germany for the treatment of liver disorders.
Papaver rhoeas	Papaveraceae	Antitussive	Many _Papaver_ alkaloids have antitussive activity.

Rhododendron fastigiatum	Ericaceae	Antiasthmatic, antispasmodic	
Althaea rosea	Malvaceae	Antileucorrheal	
Euonymus japonicus	Celastraceae	Diuretic, tonic	
Boehmeria nivea	Urticaceae	Hemostatic	
Thevetia peruviana	Apocynaceae	Congestive heart failure	Contains cardiac glycosides.
Lepidium lepidium	Cruciferae	Congestive heart failure	
Adonis amurensis	Ranunculaceae	Congestive heart failure	Contains cardiac glycosides.

Nanking College of Pharmacy Medicinal Plant Garden

After our visit to the Nanking College of Pharmacy, we drove to the outskirts of Nanking to visit the medicinal plant garden. This garden is under the management of the Department of Pharmacognosy of the College of Pharmacy. We did not receive the usual briefing prior to our visit to the garden, but presumably the previously mentioned functions for the Peking Experimental Plantation also hold true for the Nanking Medicinal Plant Garden. The Nanking garden was perhaps one third the size of the Peking facility but was laid out in about the same manner. In neither case did there appear to be any specific organization for the plants; that is, the plots were not arranged to contain plants on either a taxonomic or use basis. Again, the plants were very well taken care of, and a high degree of expertise must be attributed to those responsible for the maintenance of this facility. There was some building construction going on. In most cases, the same plants were found here as in the Peking garden. Listed below are the few plants that yielded new information.

Plant Name	Family	Use	Comments
Saponaria officinalis	Caryophyllaceae	Expectorant	Saponins known to be present in this plant would probably be the active principles.
Thalictrum fortunei	Ranunculaceae	Antipyretic	It was stated that the alkaloids were the active principle(s).

Euphorbia pekinensis	Euphorbiaceae	Cathartic	Euphorbia species are well known to have cathartic activity.
Eupatorium lindleyanum	Compositae	Antitussive	
Cannabis sativa	Cannabaceae	Analgesic	Most of the C. sativa cultivated in China is used as a source of fiber for rope. We observed hundreds of acres of this plant under cultivation in many parts of the rural countryside.

Kwangtung Provincial Botanical Garden

During our visit to Canton, we visited this most impressive botanical garden, the largest of any seen on our trip. In an introductory session, the functions of the botanical garden were stated to be

a. To introduce and cultivate plants

b. To propagate plants

c. To produce plants for research purposes

d. To supply medicinal-plant research material

e. To act as a teaching facility for pharmacy students

The area of the botanical garden was approximately 500 acres, with about 3,000 species under cultivation. It was indicated that for general use most medicinal plants were collected in the wild, but a few were cultivated. On several previous occasions, we had been told by medical workers that the preparations of Chinese herbs used as medicines were nontoxic and virtually free from side effects, but at this facility we were told that about 10 percent of medicinal plants were considered toxic and should be used with caution. This latter statement seems much more reasonable. (A member of the delegation promptly confirmed the putative toxicity of one plant by chewing a leaf, with dramatic and instant effect.)

There were about 120 workers employed at this facility. Many of the medicinal plants were arranged throughout the garden in single pots, with few growing in sufficient quantity to serve any purpose other than teaching. The botanists at this garden were extremely knowledgeable not only about the medicinal uses of the various plants but about the chemistry of certain plants now under investigation in the West. The Latin binomials were correct and up-to-date, except for a few spelling errors. Listed below are some of the plants seen and their medicinal uses in China.

Plant Name	Family	Use	Comments
Terminalia chebula	Combretaceae	Sore throat	
Ilex rubra	Aquifoliaceae	Stomach pains	
Kigelia pinnata	Bignoniaceae	Dysentery, diarrhea	
Oroxylum indicum	Bignoniaceae	Tonsillitis, diuretic	
Melia toosendan	Meliaceae	Anthelmintic	
Dalbergia hainanensis	Leguminsoae	Analgesic	
Equisetum debile	Equisetaceae	"To clarify the sight"	
Thalictrum simplex	Ranunculaceae	Antipyretic	
Dysosma chengii	Berberidaceae	Snakebite, cancer	
Stephania sinica	Menispermaceae	Analgesic, anti-inflammatory	
Urginea scilla	Liliaceae	Cardiotonic	Known to contain cardiotonic glycosides.
Acorus calamus	Araceae	Antirheumatic, snakebite	
Crinum asiaticum var. sinicum	Amaryllidaceae	Carbuncles	
Dianthus superbus	Caryophyllaceae	Diuretic	
Mirabilis jalapa	Nyctaeinaceae	Antidiabetic	
Croton crassifolius	Euphorbiaceae	Traumatic injuries	
Euphorbia sieboldiana	Euphorbiaceae	Edema (poisonous)	

Dichroa febrifuga	Saxifragaceae	Antimalarial	Known to contain febrifugine, an active principle.
Veratrum nigrum	Liliaceae	Analgesic	
Scutellaria barbata	Labiatae	Anticancer	
Aloe zebria	Liliaceae	Anti-hemmorhagic, cathartic	*Aloe* species are known to contain cathartic anthraquinones.
Euonymus chinensis	Celastraceae	Traumatic injuries	
Ventilago leiocarpa	Rhamnaceae	Antirheumatic	
Rhamnus crenatus	Rhamnaceae	Hepatitis, hepatic cirrhosis	
Datura metel	Solanaceae	Asthma, snakebite	*Datura* species are known to have antiasthmatic active principles.
Isotoma longiflora	Campanulaceae	Anticancer, snakebite, local anesthetic	
Symphytum officinale	Boraginaceae	To promote circulation, anti-inflammatory	Known to contain allantoin, which has anti-inflammatory activity.
Senecio scandens	Compositae	Skin sores, anti-inflammatory	
Elephantopus tomentosus	Compositae	Postpartum headache, anti-inflammatory, tonsillitis	
Zanthoxylum nitidum	Rutaceae	Analgetic, antirheumatic	
Zanthoxylum dissitum	Rutaceae	Analgetic, antirheumatic	

Tylophora ovata	Asclepiadaceae	Anticancer	Known to contain alkaloids such as tylophorine that have anticancer activity.
Cymbidium sp.	Orchidaceae	Respiratory stimulant	
Pholidota chinensis	Orchidaceae	Antitussive	
Dendrobium aggregatum	Orchidaceae	Antitussive	
Haemaria discolor	Orchidaceae	Tuberculosis	
Begonia crassiostus	Begoniaceae	Anticancer, for hepatitis	*Begonia* species have been shown to have *in vitro* anticancer activity.
Nepenthes mirabilis	Nepenthaceae	Antihypertensive, jaundice	
Polypodium vulgare	Polypodiaceae	Dissolve urinary bladder stones	
Alocasia odora	Araceae	Toxic, pneumonia, tuberculosis	

Medicinal Plant Garden of the Kwangtung Traditional Medical College, Canton

This medical college has a small medicinal plant garden containing individual specimens of about 400-500 different species growing in pots. These were well kept up, and the garden was divided into two sections, one in which the plants were arranged taxonomically and the other in which they were arranged by medical use. The garden was used primarily for teaching purposes; medical students were required to be able to identify the most important medicinal plants (stated to number 450).

In the medical college there was an extensive collection of preserved specimens of medicinally useful natural products, and apparently the medical students were required to familiarize themselves with about 600 of these. Included were not only plant materials, but snakes, sea shells, insects, fungi, minerals, and animal horns (charcoal prepared from human hair is taken orally as a hemostatic). Most of the uses for the plants seen at this facility were previously documented.

It should be pointed out that in the efforts of the Chinese to achieve self-sufficiency, a number of active principles that are used in medicine are being extracted from plants. A few statements can be made about the most important of these:

Camptotheca acuminata (Nyssaceae).

Camptothecin is extracted from this tree on a large-scale basis and is prepared in ampuls (as the sodium salt); it is said to be of some use, in conjunction with other drugs, for the treatment of stomach cancer. The seeds contain the highest concentration of camptothecin, which is used with other drugs mainly in an attempt to reduce its toxicity. Camptothecin may be administered prior to surgery.

Catharanthus roseus (Vinca rosea) (Apocynaceae).

Vincristine was stated to be used extensively in the treatment of many forms of cancer, in combination chemotherapy. One clinician indicated that the vincristine is extracted from plants grown in China. Two botanists in the North were queried about the abundance of C. roseus in China, and both indicated that it was not very abundant. On the other hand, two botanists in the South of China indicated that the plant grew in abundance in the southern part of China. It was further stated that the whole plant was used for the production of vincristine. Since vincristine is obtained in yields of about 30 g from 15 tons of C. roseus leaves (the roots and stems are devoid of this alkaloid), it does not appear that the Chinese are really extracting this alkaloid for two reasons:

1. Virtually every bit of soil suitable for the growth of plants that we observed in China was under cultivation with food plants. Catharanthus roseus would require similar soil for proper growth. It does not appear logical that the amount of land required to produce hundreds of tons of plants for the extraction of vincristine would be assigned to this purpose.
2. Because of the low yield of vincristine from C. roseus leaves, it is necessary to process at least 100,000 kg at a time in order to recover a reasonable yield of the alkaloid. Since the leaves of this plant represent only about 10 percent of the total dry weight of the plant, about 900,000 kg of dried plant would need to be processed in a single batch. Not only is it unlikely that quantities of plant material of this magnitude are available in China, but the equipment required to process this quantity of plant material probably does not exist.

It is more reasonable to believe that China is purchasing vincristine from Hungary, a known supplier of this alkaloid, than that the Chinese are producing it themselves by extraction.

Claviceps microcephala (Claviceptaceae).

Claviceps microcephala was found growing on the grass Calamagrostis epegous. It was the best of many Claviceps species for the production of ergonovine. This fungus is grown on a wheat (Triticum vulgare) substrate for 22 days to give a yield of 0.1 percent of total alkaloids, or 0.02 percent of ergonovine. However, for commercial production, a 9-day fermentation yields similar results in 1,000-liter fermentation tanks.

Rauvolfia Species.

Several indigenous *Rauvolfia* species have yielded quantities of reserpine sufficient to meet China's needs for this alkaloid.

Leguminous Seeds.

Several leguminous seeds, especially *Mucuna* species, are known to contain large amounts of L-dopa, which is used in China for the treatment of Parkinsonism. No specific plant names were mentioned, but we were told that China's needs of L-dopa were being met by extraction from plant sources.

PHARMACY AND PHARMACEUTICAL MANUFACTURING IN CHINA

Pharmacy Practice

The dispensing of drugs and other functions reserved for community and hospital pharmacists in the United States and most Western countries are carried out in a different way in the People's Republic of China.

In the community we found some pharmacies totally devoted to traditional drugs and others where Western drugs predominated. We have no data on the number of pharmacies throughout the country but were told in Canton that there are about 1,000 pharmacies serving 2.5 million people. In the United States 1,000 pharmacies would serve, on the average, 4.4 million people. Considering the fact that many, if not most, prescriptions are filled in outpatient pharmacies in hospitals, one might assume that the local pharmacies in the cities are dispensing a large volume of over-the-counter preparations. This is discussed further below.

The people working in the community pharmacies have usually had no formal university level training and have learned to prepare prescriptions and to prescribe medicines by apprenticeship for varying periods of time (from 6 months to 3 years). The preceptor in the traditional pharmacy, where only herbal preparations are sold, is the Chinese traditional doctor who also learned his trade through apprenticeship. He should not be confused with the formally trained Chinese traditional physician who practices medicine in clinics and hospitals.

We visited a traditional pharmacy in Canton briefly during lunch hour in an attempt to have an herbal prescription filled. Two of the four ingredients were unavailable and we were told that we would be able to get them only at a hospital. The young woman who waited on us said that she had apprenticed to the old master who was in charge of the shop. They had many herbs available in loose form and many ready-made dosage forms of herbal mixtures for a variety of conditions.

We also stopped at a shop that sold Western drugs and found many items for sale over the counter that would require a prescription in the United States. Some antibiotics and all narcotic drugs are apparently restricted to use by prescription only.

An important factor in current pharmacy practice is the widespread use of traditional drugs. As a result of the Cultural Revolution, usage of traditional drugs has markedly increased. More traditional doctors are being trained, including many who are already doctors of Western medicine;

research on herbal drugs seems to have increased support; and mass movements have been organized to collect new herbs.

The dispensing of outpatient herbal prescriptions is carried out, in the hospitals we visited, by individuals who would be classified in the United States as pharmacy aides or pharmacy technicians. Since there is no private practice of medicine, every hospital sees many outpatients each day, and most of them receive prescriptions. In most hospitals virtually all of these are dispensed from the hospital pharmacy's outpatient department. In some places, however, prescriptions are dispensed by local pharmacies in the community, probably due to the limited capacity of the hospital pharmacy.

A young dispensing technician at Lung Hua hospital in Shanghai said that she had been trained on the job for 18 months. Some technicians, she said, go to a special school for training in Chinese traditional herbs after completing high school. (In China a high school is referred to as a "middle school.") This was the only reference we heard to such a school and perhaps represented a misinterpretation in translation.

Herbal prescriptions are filled by weighing the correct amount of each herb on a hand-held balance and dividing it by eye into the required number of doses. Each "dose," consisting of the mixture of herbs, is wrapped in a paper sack and presented to the patient. On the sack there may be instructions for the patient's use. The patient prepares a decoction from the mixture by boiling the drugs with water for 15 minutes, straining off the liquid and boiling with a second portion of water for 40 minutes. (These amounts of time varied with different informants on other visits; perhaps there is also some individualization of instructions for different herbs.) The two liquids are combined and constitute a single day's dose, which may be divided into two portions to be taken morning and evening. Fresh decoctions must be prepared daily since there is little refrigeration in China, and the prescriptions are subject to decomposition.

Of some interest are the units used in prescribing herbal drugs. The main unit is the liang, which is equivalent to about 31.2 g. Ten ch'ien equal 1 liang and 10 li equal 1 ch'ien. A typical prescription for Ching Hung, a preparation used to treat acute appendicitis, is

Rx *Rheum tanguticum*	6 chien
Sargentodoxa cuneata	2 liang
Magnolia officinalis	3 li
Taraxacum mongolicum	1 liang

Divide into 3 doses

This preparation, incidentally, was also available as a tablet made of powdered extracts of the drugs in one hospital and as a decoction in another hospital. The physicians in the latter institution told us that they prefer the decoction because it is absorbed better. This was the only reference to bioavailability that we heard on our trip.

Because of the large volume of herbal prescriptions, the process of mixing herbs has been automated in the Peking Municipal Hospital of Chinese Traditional Medicine. There a fascinating and noisy Rube Goldberg-like machine has been built by the staff, through which, at the touch of a button on a console, a weighed quantity of herb (or herbs) is delivered to a pan. There are 240 drugs stored in the machine. Some drugs, because of their physical nature, cannot be dispensed by this machine and are added by hand. Needless to say, this machine speeds the dispensing process considerably. For example, at this hospital about 1,000 prescriptions per day (of a total of 1,400-1,500) are prepared using this machine. A similar machine was seen in operation at a relatively large traditional pharmacy on a major shopping street in Peking, and there are others in use in China.

There has been considerable discussion in the United States about automation replacing pharmacists in the mechanical dispensing function. The machine discussed above could easily be adapted for tablets and capsules, thus relieving highly trained pharmacists for other duties.

After seeing this device, it was surprising not to find such a machine at a busy place like Lung Hua Hospital in Shanghai, where about 4,000 prescriptions per day were being dispensed by hand.

There is apparently a considerable sale of herbal drugs over the counter (OTC). In a drug store in Peking, one member of the delegation asked the clerk for a good cold remedy and was shown three products, each a cylindrical tube of 12 tablets composed of a mixture of powdered extracts from herbs. All had been made in a factory in Peking and each cost about 8 cents. One of them was called Mulberry-*Chrysanthemum* Cold Tablet. Directions for use were to take 4-8 tablets twice daily with warm water. The indications on the package were "fever, cold, dizziness, coughing, lethargy and sore throat."

We also purchased a pill for headache containing extracts from three plants plus gypsum; these plants were: *Ligusticum wallichi*, *Angelica dahurica*, and *Schizonepeta tenuifolia*. This preparation was also useful for dizziness and stuffy nose, according to the label.

We noticed a large stock and variety of these OTC preparations in drug stores and in drug counters of major department stores in Peking and Shanghai. It is not possible to comment on the use of these preparations in rural areas, where the people depend on clinics in communes for primary care.

In hospitals, drugs for inpatients seem to be dispensed from floor stock. We did see the drug cabinets in several places and noted extensive stocks of Western medicines as well as herbal preparation. Generic names are usually used for Western drugs, but in one place we noted that the floor stock bottles were labeled with U.S. trade names (with the generic name in parentheses), such as Librium, Inderal, Miltown, Probanthine.

In Lung Hua Hospital in Shanghai we visited a room where decoctions were being prepared for inpatients at the rate of about 150 per day. These are prepared from individual prescriptions for herb mixtures sent from the pharmacy. There are 30 pots available and four workers (wearing surgical masks) are involved. The finished decoctions are sent to the wards in individual thermos bottles for each dose for each patient.

Pharmacy Research

China has adopted most useful Western drugs and has presumably needed pharmacists to develop dosage forms of these agents and processes to manufacture these dosage forms. There is also a considerable effort being made in the development and manufacture of new dosage forms of herbal drugs to replace the decoctions, which are inconvenient to prepare and often taste bad.

We did not visit a factory manufacturing Western drugs, but, from reports of previous U.S. visitors, we learned that China is now self-sufficient in making enough drug products to meet its own people's needs and is even exporting some drug products to Africa and Southeast Asia. We did see a small production unit in the Department of Organic Chemistry and Biochemistry at Peking University. Drugs such as ketamine, metaraminol, and polymyxin were being produced at what would be considered a pilot-plant scale. By our standards, this is a relatively primitive pharmaceutical production operation, although one cannot but admire the zeal with which the staff of the University developed this facility.

We noted in our visits that the development of dosage forms of herbal drugs is conducted by pharmacists in hospitals, universities, and factories. At the Institute of Chinese Materia Medica in Peking, for example, one of the four sections is totally devoted to development of dosage forms for herbal drugs.

It seems that China is intent on an increased emphasis on herbal drugs while at the same time not overlooking new developments in Western drugs. This emphasis is in accord with current political thought as expressed in Chairman Mao's statements regarding self-reliance and maximum use of China'a resources, the "treasure house" represented by Chinese traditional drugs, and combining Western and traditional medicine to gain the most from each.

There is a multipronged research approach being made to make better use of herbal drugs that includes:

Finding new Chinese herbs that have pharmacologic activity

Improving methods of cultivation

Isolating constituents that may have pharmacologic acitvity

Developing methods for pharmacologic screening of potentially active constituents

Improving older classical combinations of traditional drugs by eliminating ingredients found to be unnecessary

Developing modern dosage forms of traditional drugs

As mentioned above, pharmacists are heavily involved in the last item above and in analytic control work. In the future, as new active constituents are found and as more traditional drugs are used, there will probably be an even greater need for personnel to develop suitable dosage forms. We observed little, if any, attention to the many factors involved in this work in the

United States (such as drug dissolution and bioavailability, stability testing, and biopharmaceutics and pharmacokinetics). Apparently, principal attention is being paid to "turning out the products" and to manufacturing technology.

The world scientific literature seems to be available to the Chinese pharmacists and scientists. We noted, for example, in the library of the Chinese Academy of Medical Sciences, located at the Capital Hospital in Peking, recent issues of the Journal of the American Pharmaceutical Association, the American Journal of Hospital Pharmacy, and other periodicals from the United States and other Western countries. Although present priorities do not encourage full utilization of foreign technology, the necessity for improved standards of dosage form stability and biopharmaceutic performance will undoubtedly become more appreciated in the future.

There is some question about whether the current educational programs for pharmacists will be adequate to provide personnel able not only to utilize fully the Western literature but also to develop their own technical innovation in dosage form development.

Pharmacy Education

The education of the "pharmacist" is geared to a developmental function. We visited the Nanking College of Pharmacy, one of two freestanding colleges of pharmacy in the country. The other is at Shenyang. (There are also three faculties of pharmacy in medical colleges in Peking, Shanghai, and Chengtu.)

At the Nanking school the curriculum is now 3 years, as opposed to 5 years prior to the Cultural Revolution. Students study either "pharmacy" or "pharmaceutical chemistry." Graduates of the latter specialty work in factories, on chemical synthesis of drugs, and presumably on isolation of principles from herbs. Those completing the pharmacy program also work in factories and drug-control laboratories and work on dosage form development and chemical analysis.

As is true in all school curricula since the Cultural Revolution, great emphasis is placed on integrating theory with practice. At the Nanking school students and teachers go to factories to learn about practical problems, and these are used as a basis for student projects.

While this type of activity is probably beneficial in terms of training students to meet immediate needs, one might speculate that the sacrifice of basic science learning will inhibit development of the individual's abilities to grasp and utilize new concepts in the future and to do the kind of research that will lead to innovation. The educational approach is similar to that prevalent in the United States about 30 years ago, when industrial pharmacists rarely had any graduate training and were generally engaged in empiric dosage form development, which could often be better classified as "art" rather than science.

Today pharmacists in industry in the United States are generally trained at the M.S. and Ph.D. levels and are involved in basic studies related to dosage form design, manufacture, and testing, based on the advances of the past two decades in physical pharmacy, pharmacokinetics, and biopharmaceutics.

Pharmaceutical Manufacturing

Our view of pharmaceutical manufacturing in China came primarily from a visit to the Shanghai No. 2 Pharmaceutical Factory of Chinese Traditional Drugs. Here a staff of 470 produce over 30 products, using herbs and animal products as raw materials. One dosage form used for asthma, for example, was granules made from a concentrated fluid extract of an herbal mixture mixed with sucrose. The granules are packaged in "unit-dose" plastic bags, the contents of which are dissolved in hot water by the patient to make a "tea."

Tablet manufacture utilized high-speed rotary presses. It was difficult to determine from our discussion which adjuvants were used in tablet formulation, but apparently starch was included in the formula and talc was used as lubricant. Many tablet products are sugarcoated, using the usual pan-coating process, to obscure the bitter taste of the herbs. There seemed to be little concern for stability problems, and, since there were no observed valid chemical tests to detect loss of activity, we guessed that only physical changes (if anything) are used as indicators of stability.

The factory also produces at least one pill formulation and a number of liquid products and injectables. The injectables are generally made by extraction of the plant, or mixture of plants, with alcohol, removal of solvent, and dissolution of the extract in water, followed by filtration and final sterilization in ampuls.

Some oral liquid products were obviously for over-the-counter use as general tonics. We noted that some were labeled in English as well as in Chinese and were presumably for export to Southeast Asia. These resembled some of the products sold and promoted for a broad range of ills in the United States prior to Food and Drug legislation. It is extremely doubtful that the Chinese nostrums we saw would meet the proof-of-efficacy standards in the United States today. One of their products, a liquid named "Wan Nian Chun Jin," was labeled (in English):

> A tonic wine of high quality, made of valuable herbs through a scientific process, distinguished by its bright red color and limpidity, smooth mellow taste and delightful fragrance. Valuable for treatment of general debility, it serves as a carminative and nutrient for liver and kidney, helping blood circulation and strengthening sinew and bone.
>
> Directions: Regular use is recommended in any quantity desired.

Conclusions

With the expanding use of both herbal and Western drugs in China, the need for pharmacists in the development and manufacture of drug dosage forms will grow. The present status of dosage form research is not very scientific, and there is a need to educate pharmacists who can apply modern pharmaceutics (physical pharmacy and biopharmaceutics) to dosage form design.

The shortening of the curriculum in schools of pharmacy may inhibit such an effort and limit the abilities of graduates to interpret and utilize the pharmaceutics literature from the Western world, where considerable progress has been made in the past 20 years.

It would be useful for future delegations from China to the United States to learn something about modern drug dosage form development by visiting both manufacturers and schools of pharmacy. When it is possible to exchange individual scientists for longer study periods, Chinese pharmacy would benefit greatly by having individuals study pharmaceutics. Translation of modern Western texts in physical pharmacy, biopharmaceutics, and pharmaceutical analysis would be a useful project.

In the area of pharmacy practice relating to drug distribution, pharmists in China seem to be involved in only a supervisory role in hospitals, with trained dispensing technicians doing most of the actual prescription work. In the United States there is also a trend toward the use of technicians in dispensing in order to relieve the highly trained pharmacist for other activities that better utilize his training, e.g., providing drug information, and monitoring therapy for drug interactions.

At present, the latter kinds of activities do not appear to be emphasized in China. However, as the Western drugs come into more widespread use and as herbal active constituents are substituted for the crude plants, it may be expected that the incidence of adverse drug reactions will increase. Better dissemination of new information on the clinical use of drugs and more careful monitoring of drug usage will perhaps come to be recognized as necessary. Someone will have to be trained to fill this gap. This will probably not be the pharmacist in China but rather a type of "clinical pharmacologist" or "clinical pharmacist." Also, one can foresee a need for more stringent controls restricting the sale of drugs. Delegations from China to the United States might find it useful to visit one or more of the Drug Information Centers which have come into being in recent years.

In research on plant drugs aimed at discovery of new constituents, the most productive approach requires that screening for pharmacologic activity be closely integrated with the extraction and fractionation process. It would be useful in China to develop laboratories devoted to pharmacologic screening similar to those of the major U.S. pharmaceutical companies, which screen thousands of new chemical entities each year. Perhaps, in time, cooperative efforts in this area might be undertaken by our two countries.

DRUG CONTROL IN CHINA

Accustomed as our delegation was to the rigid control of drug testing, development, approval, and manufacture by the FDA, we expected to find some analogue in the Chinese Drug Control Bureau in the Ministry of Health. We found none.

Our delegation had a special meeting at night in our hotel with a leading member of the Medical Policy Bureau of the Ministry of Public Health. We had requested the meeting on several occasions during the trip in order to find out more about ministerial control of drug testing and production, but the evening failed to clarify matters.

Some members of our group later expressed the opinion that this was merely a matter of talking to the wrong person in the Ministry. The alternative explanation, to which most of use subscribed, is that the Ministry only confirmed what had already been suggested at much lower levels in a relatively informal way. By questioning cadre and technicians throughout our trip, we were later able to get some sense of this process. At the Chinese Institute of Materia Medica in Peking, for instance, we asked if there was an office or standing committee in the Ministry of Health to organize the development of a given drug. There was a drug administration within the Ministry, we were told, but it mainly enforced quality control. The decision to develop a drug was made by an ad hoc "identification" or "verification" committee (chien-ting hui) composed of representatives from the Institute, clinics, factories, and the ministries of health and of chemical industry. The impression conveyed was that of a fluid, back-and-forth coordination among different units.

The same question was pursued at the Shanghai Institute of Materia Medica. The answer was that such work is coordinated by a local coordinating group (hsieh-tsuo tsu) which is a three-in-one task force (factories, hospitals, institutes) organized to combat a specific disease. It was the bronchitis committee, for instance, that decided to develop rorifone. This was not the same as a "verification committee," that decides to move into actual production. The original coordinating group can decide to move ahead with production at the provincial level only, and the verification committee is for use on a national scale. In any case, we were struck by the degree of lower-level coordination in China today, as well as by the way (and the analogy applies to factory work as well) participants see the entire process as well as their own part in it.

The fluidity was also borne out by discussions at Lung Hua Hospital in Shanghai. In response to a question about drug development, the doctors there answered that there are two levels of development. At the lower or local level, hospitals can decide to test drugs clinically and may actually manufacture them for their own use. This practice spreads locally, and other research and clinical units may then send people to "exchange experiences." Thus a hospital in Peking might at this relatively informal level coordinate and use a drug developed in Shanghai. The "verification" level is formal and means national recognition of this process.

It would seem then that under these circumstances it is much easier for a Chinese research unit to clinically test and develop a new drug than it is for an American drug company forced to comply with FDA regulations. In the Chinese case, of course, Maoist politics again make this possible. If traditional herbal medicine is "a great treasure," developed over two millennia of folk use, then it can hardly be viewed as containing toxic elements - at least not in sufficient strength in herbal decoctions to threaten serious harm. Of course, extractions from such a decoction might prove toxic, and Chinese pharmacologists certainly are aware of that possibility. But their testing on animal models and humans is probably less controlled than American procedures because of the underlying assumption that Chinese traditional medicines as such are beneficial if properly used.

The question of drug control was explained most clearly by a medical cadre during an automobile ride in Nanking. We had just visited the College of Pharmacy, where it had been explained to us that many of the college's graduates went to work for drug-control bureaus (<u>yao chien-ting chi-kou</u>). The doctor was asked to explain how these bureaus functioned. They exist, he said, at the local, provincial, and national levels, reporting directly to the Ministry of Health. The drug-control bureaus (<u>yao chien-ting chi-kou</u>) are different from the verification committees (<u>chien-ting hui</u>), though both use the term <u>chien-ting</u>. The committee is a three-in-one group that brings together officials (representatives of the drug-control bureaus), technicians (clinicians and pharmacologists), and factory workers to approve the manufacture and sale of a drug. The doctor went on to say that such committees were useful because they kept the organic chemists from focusing solely on the isolation of active elements. Such elements alone might prove toxic or provoke adverse reactions. In combination, as in Chinese herbal compounds, their toxic effects were minimized while the beneficial effects increased synergistically. Thus, he claimed, the real work of the chemists was not to isolate active elements as such, but rather to help synthesize drugs or develop other sources for the compound when the original herbs were hard or expensive to obtain.

Added to the general fluidity and flexibility in this sector is the autonomy that medical workers appear to enjoy. The decision to test and develop a drug is made first at the local "coordinating" level, then eventually verified through a committee that gets the required permission for national manufacture from the Ministry of Health. Bureaucrats in the Ministry of Health more or less have to accept the subordinate committee's recommendations because they have only one weapon with which to counter such expertise. That, of course, is Mao's thought. And since Chairman Mao emphatically stresses health, the technicians in this case seem to have the last word. For instance, the personnel of the Tumor Research Institute in Peking can devote themselves to sophisticated research on the treatment of cancer - research that accords with their own individual interests as clinicians and scientists - under the

Maoist aegis of curing "high incidence diseases." They can also quickly take part in mass campaigns by sending research teams who indeed spend time in the countryside but in so doing also carry out sophisticated medical surveys to detect esophageal cancer. Their professional research interests are thus satisfied (the investigation has resulted in a paper that was presented at an international cancer conference in the fall of 1974), while at the same time they are living up to their obligations as medical workers to cure a particularly prevalent form of cancer in western Anhwei. This same group, by the way, heads the national coordinating committee for research into esophageal cancer.

At least in developmental research, the Cultural Revolution has brought certain important advantages. The stress on grass roots initiative and the decentralization of bureaucratic authority through institutions like the work conference and meetings to exchange experiences[1] has introduced a great deal of flexibility when it comes to deciding just which drugs should be developed. At first this was difficult for us to see. As one China specialist has remarked, it is best to think of the Chinese political system as

> a system of nesting boxes in which what is really going on is encased in a camouflaging organization which pretends to be where the action is. This organization is declared "absolutely top secret" and boxed in another layer of bureaucracy which is declared "top secret," and so on until you come to the outer layer, which is avowedly public and utterly ceremonial.[2]

By the end of our trip, however, many of us not only began to have a feeling for the looseness of the controls but began to wonder whether the looseness is not for China - at least for the present - superior to a U.S. FDA-type superstructure. If most of the drugs available in China are either time-tested over the centuries (and hence at least safe, in all likelihood) or drugs developed and well evaluated in many other countries prior to Chinese use, how much need is there for new clinical or toxicologic studies? We concluded that the present benevolent attitude toward drug development of both Western and traditional types was probably beneficial, although one could not help wondering what the toxic price might be for any overuse of Western chemicals.

THE VALIDATION OF CLAIMS FOR TRADITIONAL MEDICINES

To the foreigner skeptical of either the efficacy or safety of traditional medicines despite centuries of consumer satisfaction, there was little solace in a trip to China in 1974. The use of multiple drugs, often changed from day to day on an "individualistic" basis that cannot be readily explained to foreigners, and often in conjunction with Western drugs in the treatment of diseases that are notoriously unpredictable in their course - all these factors will drive a Western scientist to distraction. When a visitor notes, in addition, that serious ailments (such as cancer or cardiac dysrhythmias) are treated exclusively or primarily with Western drugs, the temptation is great to write the whole system off except as an exercise in pacifying the masses with nostrums.

Historical controls are not useful, because of past Chinese disinclination to compile statistics. Placebo-controlled trials are out, since the Chinese object to such "deception." We did hear, however, of a few tentative efforts at controlled trials, pitting traditional remedies against Western drugs. If such trials show no differences, the results will be of little use, since one cannot prove the null hypothesis, and there are many ways for a trial to miss a real difference between treatments.

But if a traditional medicine should, in a well-organized trial, prove <u>superior</u> to a standard Western drug, that would be impressive. We heard of two trials that pointed in this direction: a comparison of a traditional drug vs. Persantin for angina pectoris and one of another herbal medicine vs. dopamine for cardiogenic shock. The existence of such trials was most encouraging (although the fact that the experimental groups were grossly unequal in size made one suspicious about the "randomization").

Nor is the answer likely to lie, in the immediate future, with a search for active principles. Such research is extremely difficult and not well done in many places anywhere in the world, since chemists often isolate either that which is easy to isolate or that which is present in largest quantity - irrational touchstones for success.

More readily applicable is the use of animal systems to study crude extracts, looking for pharmacologic activity that is supportive of the attributed clinical effects. The problems here relate not only to the potential for variable pharmacologic activity in crude extracts, but also to the limited number of sensitive and specific animal analogues of human disease.

From the standpoint of documenting <u>some</u> biologic activity in herbal extracts, however, the Chinese have been successful in a number of instances.

Many issues of the Chinese Medical Journal, for example, contain articles describing laboratory research with traditional medicines. While it is not always possible to relate the recorded animal findings to the putative clinical utility, at the very least these studies show that the herbs are not pharmacologically inert. Ginseng, one of the most famous traditional plants, is used to treat so many conditions that one is tempted to think of it as an elegant placebo, but laboratory research attests to its multiple effects in biological systems.[1]

In general, the Chinese seem to be focussing primarily on clinical studies as a first step in pursuing leads supplied by traditional medicine. One cannot fault the Chinese for studying traditional drugs in man before they study them in animals. Before wasting time on laboratory attempts to explain an action or to isolate an active principle, it is imperative to know that the medicine has useful activity. And since these traditional medicines have been used on so many people for so long with apparent safety, ethical and medical fears should be minimal.

One member of our delegation, Professor Norman Farnsworth, has examined the problem of validation from another vantage point, one not available for new and untried chemicals. This includes the technique of convergent evolution. If peoples geographically distinct use a given plant for the same purpose, does that not constitute impressive *prima facie* evidence that the putative use is valid? Is not the likelihood of such a phenomenon being due to chance statistically remote?

Table A-3 in Appendix A (p.83) is an evaluation of 248 plant and animal drugs listed in a formulary-type book that was given to our delegation when we visited the Institute of Materia Medica of the Chinese Academy of Medical Sciences in Peking.[2] The book was apparently prepared by this Institute and was intended as a guide to barefoot doctors and other medical practitioners in the rural areas, to aid them in the identification of local plants that could be used as drugs and to give them the medical uses of each plant or animal. As is usual, these drugs were used in admixture with other plant and animal materials, yielding about 796 different prescriptions. Each prescription was indicated for one or more uses. The book also contains several pages of elementary botany, sufficient to familiarize the users with the terminology used for plant identification. Accurate color pictures of each plant or animal indicated in the book were included. One strange fact was our failure to see any of the combinations in this book in use in the hospitals we visited. It is possible that the book, produced to aid barefoot doctors and rural practitioners, contains medicines intended for use by paramedical personnel.

For purposes of evaluation, it was considered of importance to determine whether the prescription (usually a mixture of several ingredients) had a valid pharmacological basis, justifying its use in Chinese traditional medicine. Thus, if data were found in the literature on which a value judgment could be made to justify the use of the total prescription, the use was considered valid.

In Table A-3 the natural products are listed alphabetically by family, rather than in order of their medical uses. In the first column the family name is given, and directly below this are the species used as medicines, together with synonyms, where important. Below this, the part of the organism used in the prescription is given. In the second column, there is included a translation of the uses, the method of preparation of the prescriptions, and the additional natural products added to the prescriptions, where this was given. The third column gives an analysis of the chemical compounds found in the species indicated where they are important to the consideration of biological activities, the pharmacological activities (in man, in animals, or in vitro) for the given species, the folkloric uses for the species when this information was found for the plant outside of the People's Republic of China, and, where no data could be found on the species in question, any of the above data that could be found on other species of the genus. It was felt that on chemotaxonomic grounds, related species of a genus would generally contain similar, if not identical, chemical compounds, that could be expected to have similar or identical biological activities. Data are reported for the primary plant, followed by data on plants making up polyprescriptions. Since many of the plants were used in mixtures, the sum total of the pharmacologic effects would be of interest. Original literature references are not included in the present report.

The source of reference literature was as follows: The literature files of the Department of Pharmacognosy and Pharmacology, of the University of Illinois, contain computerized information on all chemical compounds detected in or isolated from living organisms, in addition to all pharmacological effects reported on living organisms. These data were obtained from a careful reading of each issue of Chemical Abstracts and Biological Abstracts from the year 1970 to the present. In addition, these files include most of the data on biologic acitivities from about 1964 on, and sporadically prior to that, based on needs to accumulate information for current projects. Included in the files are complete literature searches through all issues of Biological Abstracts and Chemical Abstracts on about 400 genera of plants. An asterisk was placed to the left of each primary plant in Table A-3 if the data given in the third column were derived from the analysis of references on completely searched genera of plants. While it is true that this information cannot be considered complete, it was felt that on the basis of the results presented in Table A-3 a good general analysis of most of the plants could be made.

Thus a rational basis for the alleged uses of 44.7 percent of the 796 prescriptions evaluated may exist, based on clinical results; on pharmacological evaluations of extracts of the plants in the prescriptions or of related species; or on pharmacologic effects of chemical compounds that are known to be present in the plants of the prescription or that can reasonably be predicted to exist in those plants. Another 5.3 percent of prescriptions contain species that have no confirmed pharmacologic activity but that are used for the same medical indications in a culture outside of China, and 1.3 percent contain species similar to those used for the same clinical conditions in another culture. No predictions could be made on about 48.7 percent of the plants because of a lack of interpretable data in the scientific literature. Thus it would appear that many of the 796 plants (or animals) are excellent candidates for future pharmacologic and phytochemical investigations.

In the opinion of Dr. Farnsworth, this percentage of known or predictably known useful pharmacologic effects for traditional Chinese medicines is considerably higher than would result from an analysis of medicinal plants used in the West.

Finally, it should be pointed out that the plants listed in the book that has been analyzed represent only those plants thought to be important in the Peking area. It is to be expected that other provinces could produce similar books that would describe many other medicinal plants.

BIOMEDICAL EDUCATION IN CHINA

At several different institutions, we had the opportunity to observe current Chinese thought and practice regarding the selection of students and the nature of the curricula.

The Kwangtung College of Traditional Chinese Medicine in Canton is relatively new. The building was erected in 1956 after official policy restored traditional medicine to a position equal to that of Western medicine. At present this school has 200-300 new students per year, as well as 200 Western-trained doctors who are receiving education in traditional Chinese medicine. The introductory session to the visit was exceedingly political. We heard again that the revisionists under Liu Shao-chi held the school back, but that after the Cultural Revolution there were great developments in education according to the dictates of Chairman Mao. We were told very clearly that education must serve politics. Peasants and workers are admitted in an open-door policy of education. The curriculum has been reduced from 6 to 3 years, and the number of departments has decreased. Chinese and Western medicine are combined. We were taken to a central room that contained 1,100 herbs and were told that all of these have medical activity of some sort and that in the first year of the curriculum a student has to memorize the action of some 600 of these drugs along with 150 Western ones.

We were given some details of the curriculum. The following are the units:

1. Theory of Chinese medicine and Chinese pharmacy.

2. Anatomy, physiology and biochemistry in an integrated course. Also in this segment, which is obviously the basic science segment, they include bacteriology, pharmacology, and pathology. It is not clear to what extent these were integrated.

3. The third segment, which is now in the second year, is physical diagnosis and clinical courses.

4. The medical specialties.

5 and 6. These two segments, the third year, are work in the hospital combining internal medicine and psychiatry. Some of this clinical work is done in farms, communes, and factories.

Superficially this resembles the curriculum of a Western medical school, and the length of training is the same. If during this training period the student has to grasp the very complex philosophical background of traditional medicine with its systems of humors and emphasis on hundreds of herbs, it must be an exceedingly difficult curriculum, particularly if the faculty is conscientious about integrating and "marrying" this with Western medicine. (It should be emphasized that the modern traditionally trained Chinese physician is a far cry in his training from the traditional Chinese doctor of older times, whose training was usually by apprenticeship.) We were not able to find out anything about the actual course content of the teaching of pharmacology or any basic science in this school. We saw no research, no classes, and no students; presumably, school was not in session.

As to the proportion of doctors being trained in traditional and Western medicine, we encountered different estimates - as high as one third and as low as one tenth trained in the traditional mode. From discussions with some of our Western-trained hosts, we had the impression that this emphasis on traditional medicine may be but a phase, that it will merge more and more with the Western, and that the current emphasis on herbal pharmacology will diminish as Chinese medicine ultimately combines the best of the traditional and Western schools.

On June 25 we visited Chung Shan Medical College, a Western-type school, in Canton. We were greeted by the vice-chairman of the Revolutionary Committee, Yao Ch'ung-jen, who proceeded to give us an articulate and concise explanation of the college and its post-Cultural Revolution teaching methods. He first explained that there were five hospitals affiliated with the college (itself an amalgamation of the former Chung Shan, Ling Nan, and Kuang Hua medical facilities). The college admits 600 medical students each year and also enrolls 120 nursing students. Before the Cultural Revolution, he claimed, students were admitted solely on the basis of marks. Since then, four new criteria have been adopted for matriculation: the applicants must know Mao Tse-tung's thought and Marxism-Leninism; they must have had more than 2 years of practical experience as workers, peasants, or soldiers; they must possess a "cultural level" equal to graduation from high school; and they must be about 20 years old, single, and in good health. One can believe, too, that these more mature students work a lot harder than their pre-Cultural Revolution counterparts. One recalled those days after World War II when the ex-soldiers came to U.S. college campuses under the GI Bill and delighted professors accustomed to the more usual (and less devoted) kind of student.

Dr. Yao also explained that the college operates according to the "open door" principle, following Mao's June 26 directive to stress the rural areas. The college keeps in close contact with commune hospitals to which students are sent by rotation. Moreover, mobile medical teams are sent to communes to give short training courses to barefoot doctors and other paramedical workers. (One third of the students are former "barefoot doctors.") The curriculum here, too, had been shortened from 6 to 3 years, which meant reducing a 36-course syllabus to 15 courses. As Ho Tzu-ch'ien, the leading member of the Educational Revolutionary Committee later described them, the fifteen courses consisted in the first year of <u>jen-t'i hsueh</u> (study of the human body, combining anatomy, histology, biochemistry, and physiology), parasitology, microbiology, pathology and pharmacology; in the second, of diagnostics, internal medicine, surgery, traditional medicine, gynecology and regional anatomy; and in the third, of "service by curing" (each student being given responsibility for five to ten patients), clinical pharmacology, radioisotopes, and "recent progress in medicine."

Before starting this 3-year course (classes run 6 days a week for 48 weeks each year), the incoming students are given an intensive 6-month refresher course in politics, foreign languages, mathematics, physics, and chemistry. During the formal period of study, they are also constantly kept in contact with clinical work in the society at large. The entire curriculum is designed to nurture "a spirit of independence," and by constantly combining theory and practice, makes it much easier for the students to remember what they have learned. Yao went on to explain that this new shortened curriculum was preferable to the previous 6-year one. Many courses before had been redundant, and far too much time had been spent on purely theoretical study.

Wu Hsiu-jung, a professor of pharmacology, discussed the pharmacology curriculum and the conflict between practical and theoretical subjects. The college has omitted certain matters, such as theories of anesthesia, which are certainly, to our way of thinking also, rather inconclusive. They teach some theoretical materials - for example, the effect of cardiac glycosides on calcium movements in the heart - but they stop there before it becomes too complex. They do teach a few traditional drugs, but not many. A major emphasis is placed on discussions and self-teaching. They have their own laboratory manuals. Of the total 84 hours in the first year of pharmacology, 28 hours are for laboratories and the rest for lectures. There is some clinical pharmacology later on.

In our tour of the college, we saw groups of 15 students each eagerly observing an animal experiment (really a demonstration) in physiology in which standard drugs were administered and the effects on blood pressure measured. They discussed the implications of this experiment with an instructor who used the same dialectical teaching style used in seminars in the United States. The students were eager, responsive, and quick to answer.

Peking University, founded in 1898, now has 20 departments, 75 specialties, and 2,300 teachers. After the teams of workers and People's Liberation Army cadre entered the university in 1968, as part of the Cultural Revolution, the length of study was shortened from 6 to 3 years (except for certain specialties like theoretical physics and Arabic, which now takes 4 years to complete), and productive labor was added to the curriculum. There are now seven factories (e.g., pharmaceutical plant, computer factory, and a facility for making plastics) and 27 shops on campus, each of them intimately connected with departments in the hard sciences. Students in the social sciences (humanities were not mentioned) work in factories outside the university. There is also a major difference in the kinds of students attending the university because of the new admission policies. Their "political quality" is much higher than that of earlier students, primarily because they study from a collective point of view. That is, they are sent by their unit (commune, factory, or army) to attend the university, study for it, and return to it after graduation. The student's cultural level is lower than pre-Cultural Revolution students, but their industriousness and commitment are higher.

The labs we visited were in a poor state, with inadequate or old-fashioned equipment for the most part. The few spectrometers and other machines did not seem to be in use. There were almost no students visible, most - we were told - being in the factories or with army units at the time. There were a few students in the small pharmaceutical plant, which was built by staff, students, and workers in 1969. The machinery was crude but apparently effective, and the plant made many drugs that were bottled in ampuls and packaged on site by regular (nonstudent) workers.

There is certainly merit in having the students learn about the engineering side of pharmaceutics. (One of our problems in the United States is the division of labor between pharmacists and engineers, the latter often failing to appreciate the fine points of drug manufacturing.) But time spent on this sort of manufacturing probably delays advances in pharmaceutical research. In other words, the dilemma noted by American scholars in China between pure and practical science seems a real one. On the one hand, the Chinese educational authorities are making a student's work even more relevant to the needs of society. They are injecting a heavy dose of practicality into the educational system; simply being a student is not sufficient. But at the same time they may also be depriving themselves of the capacity for higher research. Since they now take students who have attended high school, to whom they give a 6-month refresher course, and since the formal curriculum in a field like chemistry amounts to only 2 years (the third being spent in labor), university graduates have a total of only 12 years of formal schooling plus kindergarten. However, it was also pointed out that these new kinds of students are much more industrious than pre-Cultural Revolution students and they have much higher critical powers than before. But many in our group still had doubts about such students' ability to do significant research, especially once the older generation of Western-trained scientists retires. Since 1971, the university has accepted 5,600 students in regular programs and 7,000 in short courses. The first group of 2,300 under the new curriculum were graduated in January 1974.

It was less clear to us how postgraduate training is arranged for. Peking University, for example, has no formal postbaccalaureate students but does retain 150 students from each graduating class as a resevoir of candidates for instructional and research appointments.

At Chung Shan Medical College, we asked what happens to students who want to do further work in a basic science, such as pharmacology. Such students would apply to return to the department, and the department could apply to the ministry for the assignment of such students. There are no formal degrees involved in any of this, neither M.D. nor Ph.D. From that standpoint, the whole fabric of medical training and graduate training is quite unstructured.

The Institute of Chinese Materia Medica in Peking offers training and research facilities to three kinds of presumably advanced students: people with "practical experience" who are transferred from their commune, factory, or army units to receive "supplementary training" for an indeterminate length of time, university students in their last year who "enter for training" before being allocated by the government to other units, and a pool of future researchers requested by the Institute to become lifetime members. Perhaps the most important single question concerning the future of Chinese medical and pharmacological science - and of other scientific fields as well - is whether this reservoir of talent is going to be allowed to continue to accumulate and provide a successor generation. Campaigns like the one criticizing Lin Piao and Confucius, or even future movements of the intensity of the Cultural Revolution at its peak in the late '60's, could easily single out such researchers as an incipient technocratic elite. If disbanded, these pools of talent would not easily be recovered.

Assuming that significant scientific advance is the goal, it is imperative for the Chinese to keep their research institutes well staffed. It is also important that younger staff members, especially in fields like chemistry, be kept in close touch with worldwide scientific developments. Although this may render them more vulnerable to criticism from nativist movements within China, younger men and women need to break out of their cultural isolation and have greater contacts with the international scientific community. It is now the Western-trained scientists that provide much of the direction for basic research. When that group passes, the next generation should have the opportunity to continue to "exchange experiences" with other countries' scholars, either at home or abroad. Outsiders cannot impose this upon the Chinese, but we certainly can hope to work for longer-term exchanges between China and the United States. As the Chinese may benefit from whatever we can offer in the way of techniques and ideas, so may we profit from their advances and perhaps even absorb the extraordinary sense of social responsibility displayed by so many of the scientists we encountered in the course of our journey in the People's Republic of China.

The question of postgraduate training in medical specialties arose on a few occasions. We concluded that this is accomplished in an informal way. Several of the hospitals are said to do postgraduate teaching, and we saw a general surgeon from one hospital performing brain surgery under supervision at another hospital as part of his specialty training in neurosurgery. Nevertheless, the absence of truly "junior" physicians was striking at most hospitals.

GENERAL MEDICAL CARE IN CHINA

It was not our responsibility to assess the level of medical care in China. Nor could we have done it properly, in view of the specialized nature of our delegation and the places we visited. Nevertheless, we should like to pass on a few impressions about Chinese hospital medicine.

These impressions were overwhelmingly favorable. We met many intelligent and up-to-date physicians. Hospital charts usually contained results of relevant laboratory tests, the x-rays were of high quality, and the surgeons impressive. Perhaps most remarkable, however, were the more "human" aspects of medical care in China. The quality of relations between doctors and patients seemed excellent, and the spirits of the patients in the hospital remarkable. They smiled and clapped when we came in, and their good spirits certainly must be a considerable aid in their recovery.

The patients seem to know the details of their illnesses to a degree that would be unusual in the United States. Even 6-and 7-year-old children with congenital heart defects knew the technical names of their diseases and discussed their recent or forthcoming operations quite openly. We were told that this sort of frankness was absolutely required on the part of the staff. Common discussion of this sort seems not only to remove the mystery from medicine but to give patients a sense of faith and confidence.

The same frankness was tendered to terminal cancer patients in the wards we visited in Canton, wards unmarked by despair. The doctors asserted that they tell patients everything about their illnesses, including statistics about mortality, and they openly discussed every aspect of a case with us in the patient's presence. Yet the invalids' faces, manners, and words were all reasonably composed and often cheerful. The only person in apparent discomfort was a woman with uterine cancer who had just received an arterial infusion of nitrogen mustard.

Several months ago, in a letter to the editor of the New England Journal of Medicine (April 18, 1974), a Chinese-American physician, P.H. Chi-pang Wen, wrote:

> ...During a professional visit to the People's Republic of China last year, I found out that in many large teaching hospitals, as well as small rural health stations, the patient had custody of his or her own medical records. A bold-type notice in the right-upper corner on the top

page of the record clearly stated: "Take good care of this record and be sure to bring it at your next visit."

Being a socialist country stressing the egalitarian concept, China has ample reasons for this practice. The doctor-patient relation has not only been a harmonious one, but also one based on equal terms, reinforced by the recent Cultural Revolution. The medical knowledge and skill possessed by the doctor are considered a public property. Furthermore, doctors are selected and trained for their dedication to public service, and any measure that would facilitate the achievement of the goal of serving the people is encouraged and implemented. It is contended that, since the welfare of the individual patient is always in the interest of the masses, the medical record, a "vitally important part of medical care process," belongs to the masses and is subject to the scrutiny of the masses, if necessary.

To my limited observation, the practice has indeed made the system more responsive and less bureaucratic. One additional important advantage is the savings in resources and time...

CONCLUDING REMARKS

The Chinese people consume considerable quantities of herbal remedies, many of which have been in use for centuries. Both laymen and scientists subscribe to the belief that these natural products have proved their efficacy through years of consumer satisfaction and that they are extraordinarily safe. Medicines of plant, animal, and mineral origin are available both *via* prescription and "over the counter," as is true also for Western drugs. Most Western drugs appear to be available to the Chinese public, and they are the mainstays of treatment for some common and serious diseases such as cancer and cardiovascular ills. China is self-sufficient so far as the production of almost all Western drugs is concerned. We could make no assessment of any harm caused by the ready availability, without prescription, of both Western and traditional drugs.

Although there was no opportunity to evaluate the clinical effectiveness of several purified constituents isolated from Chinese traditional herbs, the following were found to be used in Chinese medicine or are currently in various stages of clinical investigation: 6-hydroxyatropine, (±)-tetrahydropalmatine and (-)-tetrahydropalmatine, neoandrographolide, (±)-tetrandrine, berberine, and esculetin. These constituents are not used in the United States and might be considered for further study of their effectiveness and safety.

A large number of traditional herbal prescriptions were observed in use in hospitals throughout the People's Republic of China. A detailed analysis of those prescriptions has been included in this report (Appendix A) and provides presumptive evidence (based on literature reports) that in many cases the prescriptions could indeed be effective for the conditions indicated. Since the active principles of these plants have in general not been isolated and identified, there is fertile ground for further investigation by natural-product chemists, pharmacognosists, and pharmacologists desirous of discovering new, biologically active compounds from plants.

Further, an analysis was made, on the basis of current literature reports, of 796 prescriptions stated to be used commonly in Chinese traditional medicine, involving 248 plant and animal products (see Appendix A). It was concluded that 44.7 percent of the prescriptions may have a rational basis for their use. Insufficient data were available in the literature to assess the value of the remaining 55.3 percent of the prescriptions. The data presented in this evaluation provide a basis for study by Western scientists to ascertain the effectiveness of unstudied plant and animal products making up these prescriptions.

Although interesting therapeutic claims are made for herbal medicines, and the above biochemotaxonomic analysis supports these contentions, we were unable, on the basis of the clinical evidence alone, to come to firm conclusions about any specific traditional drug. The reasons for this were multiple and included the unpredictable course of most symptoms or diseases, the almost total absence of controlled trials, the cultural objection to the use of placebo controls, and the simultaneous administration of multiple forms of treatment, including Western drugs.

There is no specific national plan for prescribing which of the thousands of traditional medicines should have closer clinical and laboratory scrutiny by the Chinese. That choice is often left to individual institutes following broad national guidelines. The Chinese do not have a precise analogue to our Food and Drug Administration; it is not evident that up until now the absence of such an agency has hampered China in any significant way. Whether a development in this direction will occur when the Chinese begin to produce significant numbers of new chemical drugs remains to be seen. The present policy of pursuing animal studies after clinical utility is defined for traditional medicines, while opposite to Western habits, is eminently defensible for drugs that have been used for many years with apparent safety. For new herbs not clinically studied in the past, the situation would be quite different.

The obvious politicization of student selection and curricular reform does not necessarily bode ill for Chinese science. More important, in our view, is the de-emphasis of pure research, the emphasis of developmental research, and the pejorative attitude toward scientific credentials. We feel that first-rate science and medicine require both a specialist "elite" and the opportunity to follow one's nose. Flexner's "usefulness and useless knowledge" is as valid a concept today as it was a half century ago. Current deficiencies in the number of scientific personnel and in modern techniques and equipment, attributable to the dislocations occasioned by the Cultural Revolution, will make it difficult for the Chinese to isolate new active principles.

Curriculum reform in China parallels, in many respects, curriculum reform in the United States. In both countries there is an impetus toward shortening the training period, introducing clinical contact early in the curriculum, integrating the disciplines, and emphasizing "relevance." The current selections process in China is producing a more politically conscious and perhaps more serious and dedicated type of medical student.

The marriage of traditional and Western medicine has yet to prove its durability. An empiric eclecticism now exists, rather than a full integration of the theory and practice of both systems. Despite political pressures, Western medicine is still in the ascendancy.

National priorities concerning disease states are quite similar in China and the United States. The Chinese, having more or less disposed of some major infectious disease problems, are now concentrating on bronchitis, hypertension, and cancer. This corresponds closely to our own preoccupation with cancer, heart disease, stroke, and pulmonary disease.

Perhaps the most significant impact felt by the scientific members of the delegation came from the challenge to basic assumptions long held by our own society. What we saw of acupuncture analgesia; Chinese orthopedic practices; their nonoperative approach to kidney stones, appendicitis, and perforated peptic ulcer; the geographical incidence of certain cancers; cataract surgery; burn treatment; their methods of dispensing drugs; and the respect for the opinions and experience of both patients and physicians was extremely provocative and suggested a need for Western scientists to re-examine some of their favorite dogmas.

For the future, we believe that great benefit would accrue to both China and the United States if exchanges of scientists, for prolonged periods, with opportunity for close interaction, could be arranged. In addition, we believe that Chinese pharmacologists visiting this country would profit from visits to our drug industry, the FDA, and schools of medicine. Where deficiencies in Chinese biomedical texts exist (such as, perhaps, in physiology, pharmacology, biopharmaceutics, and pharmaceutical analysis), the translation of good foreign texts would be highly desirable.

Appendix A

This appendix presents an evaluation of 248 plant and animal drugs used in the People's Republic of China. The drugs included here were listed in The Atlas of Commonly Used Chinese Traditional Drugs.*

Table A-1 lists all the plant drugs alphabetically, and Table A-2 lists all nonplant drugs. Table A-3 is the analysis of all 248 drugs; the "activity rating" included in the first column is interpreted as follows:

+5 The use in Chinese medicine can be correlated with pharmacological activities reported for the same plant in the literature, or with the known pharmacological effects of purified principles known to be present in the same plant.

+4 The use in Chinese medicine can be correlated with the pharmacological activities reported for another species of the same genus, as based on scientific reports on the pharmacological effects of crude extracts.

+3 The use in Chinese traditional medicine can be correlated with reports that the same plant is used for the same condition in countries outside of China.

+2 The use in Chinese traditional medicine can be correlated with reports that other species of the same genus are used for the same condition in countries outside of China.

0 No data, experimental or otherwise, could be found in the literature that allowed a correlation of the use of the plant in Chinese traditional medicine with other plants, the same plant, or constituents known to be present in the plant. This may be due to the fact that negative data are rarely reported in the literature, or because the plant in question, as well as related species of the same genus, have not been previously investigated for pharmacological activity.

---

*Revolutionary Committee of the Institute of Materia Medica, Chinese Academy of Medical Sciences, Peking (1970).

Note: The above statements concern the title plant in each case, or another plant in a polyprescription. The rating system is only designed to rate the use of the prescription, and not necessarily the specific title plant.

Table A-1 An Alphabetical Listing of Plant and Fungal Drugs Evaluated in Table A-3*

Genus and Species	Family
Abutilon avicennae	Malvaceae
Acalypha australis	Euphorbiaceae
Acanthopanax gracilistylus	Araliaceae
5 Achillea	Compositae
3 *Achyranthes bidentata*	Amaranthaceae
Aconitum carmichaeli	Ranunculaceae
Acorus gramineus	Araceae
Acorus pseudoacorus See *Acorus gramineus*	
Agastache rugosa	Labiatae
Agrimonia viscidula	Rosaceae
Ailanthus altissima	Simaroubaceae
Ajuga decumbens	Labiatae
5/575) Alangium chinense	Marleaceae
Alisma plantago-aquatica var. *orientale*	Alismataceae
Amblytropis multiflora	Leguminosae
Ampelopsis japonica	Vitaceae
Anemarrhena asphodeloides	Liliaceae
Anemone hupehensis var. *japonica*	Ranunculaceae
Angelica anomala	Umbelliferae
Angelica dahurica	Umbelliferae
Angelica pubescens	Umbelliferae
Angelica sinensis	Umbelliferae
Aquilaria sinensis	Thymelaeaceae
Arctium lappa	Compositae

*This table is provided to aid the reader in locating plants in Table A-3, since plants are entered in alphabetical order of their appropriate family.

Areca catechu	Palmae
Arisaema consanguineum	Araceae
Aristolochia debilis	Aristolochiaceae
Aristolochia contorta	Aristolochiaceae
Aristolochia westlandi	Aristolochiaceae
Artemisia apiacea	Compositae
Artemisia argyi	Compositae
Artemisia capillaris	Compositae
Asarum heterotropoides var. *mandshuricum*	Aristolochiaceae
Asparagus cochinchinensis	Liliaceae
Aster tataricus	Compositae
Astragalus membranaceus	Leguminosae
Atractylodes lancea	Compositae
Atractylodes macrocephala	Compositae
Baphicacanthus cusia	Acanthaceae
Berberis amurensis	Berberidaceae
Bidens bipinnata	Compositae
Bletilla striata	Orchidaceae
Broussonetia papyrifera	Moraceae
Brucea javanica	Simaroubaceae
Bupleurum falcatum var. *stenophyllum*	Umbelliferae
Bupleurum scorzoneraefolium	See *Bupleurum falcatum* var. *stenophyllum*
Callicarpa dichotoma	Verbenaceae
Campsis grandiflora	Bignoniaceae
Cannabis sativa	Cannabaceae
Capsella bursa-pastoris	Cruciferae

Carthamus tinctorius	Co[illegible]
Cassia tora	Leguminosae
Celosia argaricalea See *Celosia argentea*	
Celosia argentea	Amaranthaceae
Centipeda minima	Compositae
Cephalanopsis segetum	Compositae
Chaenomeles lagenaria	Rosaceae
Chaenomeles sinensis	Rosaceae
Changium smyrnioides	Umbelliferae
Chrysanthemum indicum	Compositae
Chrysanthemum morifolium	Compositae
Cimicifuga foetida	Ranunculaceae
Cinnamomum cassia	Lauraceae
Cirsium japonicum	Compositae
Citrus aurantium	Rutaceae
Citrus spp.	Rutaceae
Clematis chinensis	Ranunculaceae
Clematis montana	Ranunculaceae
Clerodendrum trichotomum	Verbenaceae
Codonopsis pilosula	Campanulaceae
Commelina communis	Commelinaceae
Coptis chinensis	Ranunculaceae
Cornus officinalis	Cornaceae
Corydalis bulbosa	Papaveraceae
Crataegus cuneata	Rosaceae
Crataegus pinnatifida	Rosaceae

Cuscuta chinensis	Convolvulaceae
Cyathula capitata	Amaranthaceae
Cynanchum atratum	Asclepiadaceae
Cynanchum glaucescens	Asclepiadaceae
Cynanchum stauntoni	Asclepiadaceae
Cyperus rotundus	Cyperaceae
Datura metel	Solanaceae
Dendrobium hancockii	Orchidaceae
Descurainia sophia	Cruciferae
Dichroa febrifuga	Saxifragaceae
5(578) Dicliptera japonica	Acanthaceae
Dioscorea batatas	Dioscoreaceae
Dioscorea nipponica	Dioscoreaceae
Dipsacus asper	Dipsacaceae
Dryopteris crassirhizoma	Polypodiaceae
5(576) Dysosma aurantiocaulis	Berberidaceae
Eclipta alba See Eclipta prostrata	
Eclipta prostrata	Compositae
Eclipta punctata See Eclipta prostrata	
Ephedra sinica	Ephedraceae
Equisetum hiemale	Equisetaceae
Eriobotrya japonica	Rosaceae
Eriocaulon buergerianum	Eriocaulaceae
Eucommia ulmoides	Eucommiaceae
Eupatorium fortunei	Compositae
Euphorbia humifusa	Euphorbiaceae
Euphorbia kansui	Euphorbiaceae
Evodia rutaecarpa	Rutaceae
Foeniculum vulgare	Umbelliferae
Forsythia suspensa	Oleaceae

Fraxinus rhynchophylla	Oleaceae
Fritillaria cirrhosa	Liliaceae
Fritillaria thunbergii	Liliaceae
Fritillaria verticillata See *Fritillaria thunbergii*	
Gardenia jasminoides	Rubiaceae
Gastrodia elata	Orchidaceae
Gentiana macrophylla	Gentianaceae
Gentiana scabra	Gentianaceae
Ginkgo biloba	Ginkgoaceae
Glehnia littoralis	Umbelliferae
Glycyrrhiza uralensis	Leguminosae
+*Grifola umbellata*	Polyporaceae
Gynandropsis gynandra	Capparidaceae
Gynura segetum	Compositae
Hibiscus mutabilis	Malvaceae
Hocquartia manshuriensis	Aristolochiaceae
Houttuynia cordata	Saururaceae
Hyoscyamus niger	Solanaceae
Hypericum japonicum	Guttiferae
Imperata cylindrica	Gramineae
Inula japonica	Compositae
Ipomoea hederacea	Convolvulaceae
Isatis tinctoria	Cruciferae
Knoxia corymbosa	Rubiaceae
Kochia scoparia	Chenopodiaceae
Ledebouriella seseloides	Umbelliferae
Leonurus heterophyllus	Labiatae

Lepidium apetalum	Cruciferae
Ligusticum wallichii	Umbelliferae
Ligustrum lucidum	Oleaceae
Lilium brownii var. *colchesteri*	Liliaceae
Lindera strychnifolia	Lauraceae
Lithospermum erythrorhizon	Boraginaceae
Lobelia chinensis	Campanulaceae
Lonicera japonica	Caprifoliaceae
Lophatherum gracile	Gramineae
Lycium barbarum	Solanaceae
Lycium chinense	Solanaceae
Lycopus lucidus	Labiatae
Macrotomia euchroma	Boraginaceae
Magnolia officinalis	Magnoliaceae
Malva chinensis See *Malva verticillata*	
Malva verticillata	Malvaceae
Melia toosendan	Meliaceae
Mentha arvensis	Labiatae
Morinda officinalis	Rubiaceae
Morus alba	Moraceae
Nelumbo nuciferum	Nymphaeaceae
Notopterygium incisum	Umbelliferae
Ophiopogon japonicus	Liliaceae
Paeonia lactiflora	Paeoniaceae
Paeonia suffruticosa	Paeoniaceae
Panax ginseng	Araliaceae
5(573) *Paris polyphylla*	Liliaceae
Perilla frutescens var. *crispa*	Labiatae

Periploca sepium	Asclepiadaceae
Peucedanum praeruptorum	Umbelliferae
Phellodendron amurense	Rutaceae
Phragmites communis	Gramineae
Physalis francheti var. bunyardii	Solanaceae
Phytolacca esculenta	Phytolaccaceae
Pinellia ternata	Araceae
Pinellia tuberifera See Pinellia ternata	
Plantago asiatica	Plantaginaceae
Platycodon grandiflorum	Campanulaceae
Polygala tenuifolia	Polygalaceae
Polygonatum officinale	Liliaceae
Polygonum aviculare	Polygonaceae
Polygonum chinense See Polygonum multiflorum	
Polygonum cuspidatum	Polygonaceae
Polygonum hydropiper	Polygonaceae
Polygonum multiflorum	Polygonaceae
Polygonum orientale	Polygonaceae
Polygonum pilosum See Polygonum orientale	
+Poria cocos	Polyporaceae
Portulaca oleracea	Portulacaceae
Portulaca sativa See Portulaca oleracea	
Prunella vulgaris	Labiatae
Prunus armeniaca	Rosaceae
Prunus armeniaca var. ansu	Rosaceae
Prunus mume	Rosaceae
Prunus persica	Rosaceae
Psoralea corylifolia	Leguminosae

Pteris multifida	Polypodiaceae
Pueraria lobata See Pueraria pseudo-hirsuta	
Pueraria pseudo-hirsuta	Leguminosae
Pulsatilla chinensis	Ranunculaceae
Punica granatum	Punicaceae
Pyrola rotundifolia	Pyrolaceae
Pyrrosia lingua	Polypodiaceae
Quisqualis indica	Combretaceae
Ranunculus zuccarinii	Ranunculaceae
Raphanus sativus	Cruciferae
Rauvolfia verticillata	Apocynaceae
Rehmannia glutinosa f. hueichingensis	Scrophulariaceae
Rheum tanguticum	Polygonaceae
Rosa laevigata	Rosaceae
Rubia cordifolia	Rubiaceae
Rubia munjista See Rubia cordifolia	
Rumex crispus	Polygonaceae
Rumex obtusifolium See Rumex crispus	
Rumex patientia	Polygonaceae
Salsola collina	Chenopodiaceae
Salvia miltiorhiza	Labiatae
5(577) Sambucus javanica	Caprifoliaceae
Sanguisorba officinalis	Rosaceae
Saussurea lappa	Compositae
5(574) Scheffera arboricola	Araliaceae
Schisandra chinensis	Schisandraceae
Schizonepeta tenuifolia	Labiatae
Scrophularia ningpoensis	Scrophulariaceae
Scutellaria baicalensis	Labiatae
Selaginella tamariscina	Selaginellaceae

Semiaquilegia adoxoides	Ranunculaceae
Sesamum indicum	Pedaliaceae
Siegesbeckia pubescens	Compositae
Solanum americanum See Solanum nigrum	
Solanum nigrum	Solanaceae
5(572) Solidago virgo-aurea L.	Compositae
Sonchus brachyotus	Compositae
Sophora flavescens	Leguminosae
Sophora japonica	Leguminosae
Sophora subprostrata	Leguminosae
Sparganium stoloniferum	Sparganiaceae
Spatholobus suberectus	Leguminosae
Stemona sessilifolia	Stemonaceae
5(570) Stephania tetrandra	Menispermaceae
Tamarix chinensis	Tamaricaceae
Taraxacum mongolicum	Compositae
Tetrapanax papyriferum	Araliaceae
Thuja orientalis	Cupressaceae
Tribulus terrestris	Zygophyllaceae
Trichosanthes kirilowii	Cucurbitaceae
Trichosanthes multiloba	Cucurbitaceae
Tussilago farfara	Compositae
Typha latifolia	Typhaceae
Typhonium giganteum	Araceae
Uncaria rhynchophylla	Rubiaceae
Vaccaria pyramidata	Caryophyllaceae
Valeriana stubendorfi	Valerianaceae
Viscum coloratum	Loranthaceae
Xanthium strumarium	Compositae

Zizyphus _jujuba_ var. _spinosa_ Rhamnaceae

Zizyphus _mauritiana_ See _Zizyphus_ _jujuba_ var. _spinosa_

+Fungi.

Table A-2. A List of Animal and Other Non-Plant Drugs Evaluated in Table A-3

Scientific name	Common name
Agkistrodon acutus	Snake
Allolobophora caliginosa	Earthworm
Bombyx mori	Silkworm
Bos taurus domesticus	Ox
Buthus martensi	Scorpion
Chinemys reevesii	Tortoise
Cryptotympana atrata	-
Eupholyphaga sinensis	-
Gallus gallus domesticus	Chicken
Gekko gecko	Lizard
Haliotis diversicolor	Abalone
Hierodula spp.	-
Hirudo nipponica	Leech
Lamprotula leai	-
Ostrea spp.	Oyster
Scolopendra subspinipes mutilans	Centipede
Sepia esculenta	Cuttlefish
Trogopterus xanthipes	-
Whitmania pigra	-
Sodium sulfate	

TABLE A-3 ANALYSIS OF 248 PLANT AND ANIMAL DRUGS USED IN THE PEOPLE'S REPUBLIC OF CHINA[a]

DRUG[b]	USE	ANALYSIS
ACANTHACEAE		
√*Baphicacanthus cusia* Dried root, rhizomes and leaves	a. Same uses as for *Isatis tinctoria* (Cruciferae).	Nothing of value was found in the literature regarding *B. cusia*. *Isatis tinctoria* has been shown to have antibacterial properties *in vitro*.
Activity Rating = +5,+5		

[a]Drugs listed here are those listed in *The Atlas of Commonly Used Chinese Traditional Drugs*, Revolutionary Committee of the Institute of Materia Medica, Chinese Academy of Medical Sciences, Peking (1970).

[b]For an interpretation of the activity rating, see p. 80.

ALISMATACEAE

✓ Alisma plantago-aquatica var. orientale.

Dried tubers

a. For edema, dysuria and venereal disease, decoct with Plantago asiatica, Poria cocos and Grifola umbellata.

b. For "kidney weak" type of vertigo, lumbago, and premature ejaculation, decoct with Rehmannia glutinosa, Cornus officinalis and Paeonia suffruticosa.

Alisma plantago-aquatica is famous in Chinese medicine as a remedy for hypertension, diabetes and nephritis, although these are not all indicated in the prescriptions being considered. A large amount of work has centered around the investigation of the serum cholesterol lowering constituents of this plant, and the active constituent has been identified as a novel triterpene, alisol A. Extracts of this plant have also shown anti-cancer activity, as has the related species, A.brevipes. Extracts have also been shown effective in repairing carbon tetrachloride induced fatty liver degeneration, and they have been shown to produce hypoglycemia in animals. Paeoniflorin from Paeonia albiflora, has been shown to elicit anit-inflammatory activity, thus partially explaining the uses in prescription (b).

Activity Rating = 0,+4

AMARANTHACEAE

√Achyranthes bidentata

Dried root

a. Use raw as a coagulant.
b. Use in tincture form as a tonic.
c. For weakness (impotency), lumbago and pains in the knees and joints. Decoct with Rehmannia glutinosa, Dipsacus aspera, Cuscuta chinensis and Psoralea corylifolia.
d. For amenorrhea, epistaxis and toothache, decoct with Ophiopogon japonicus, Anemarrhena asphodeloides and Angelica sinensis.
e. For anxiety, thirst, headache and toothache, decoct with Rehmannia glutinosa, Ophiopogon japonicus, Anemarrhena asphodeloides and calcium sulfate.

Achyranthes bidentata has been used as an herbal remedy outside of China as a diuretic and antipyretic, however no direct information could be found in the literature relative to the chemical constituents or pharmacological activities of this species. On the other hand, Achyranthes species appear to be rather chemically homogeneous, and from information reported from related species, one can speculate that Achyranthes bidentata would be chemically and pharmacologically similar to the related species. An uncharacterized saponin from Achyranthes aspera has shown cardiac stimulant activity, and achyranthine, an uncharacterized alkaloid from A. aspera, has been shown to decrease blood pressure and heart rate, dilate blood vessels, and increase the rate and amplitude of respiration in dogs and in frogs. The contractile effect of the alkaloid on frog rectus abdominis muscle was less than that of acetylcholine and its spasmogenic effect was not blocked by tubocurarine. Achyranthine had diuretic and purgative activities in rats. The alkaloid showed no effects on isolated guinea pig and rat ileum, or on the central nervous system, nor did it have any irritant effect on the rabbit ear and cornea, but had a slight antipyretic activity in rats. Ecdysterone and inokosterone, two steroidal insect moulting hormones present in most *Achyranthes* species, stimulate protein synthesis in mouse liver cells. An extract of *Achyranthes aspera* was shown to be hypertensive, cardiotonic and to relax intestinal muscle. *Achyranthes aspera* has been used, with some degree of success, in extract form, for the treatment of human leprosy. The ecdysones present in this plant have shown effectiveness in humans as analgesics.

Activity Rating = 0,0,+5,+5,0

Celosia argentea (Syn. *Celosia argaritacea*)

Dried ripe seed

a. For "liver fire", ophthalmia, photophobia and headache, decoct with *Morus alba*, *Chrysanthemum morifolium*, *Equisetum hiemale* and *Gentiana scabra*.
b. For "fogged eye", "blurred eye", decoct with *Eriocaulon buergerianum*.

Celosia argentea (*C.argaritacea*) has folkloric uses outside of China as an aphrodisiac and for cancer. Experimentally it has been shown to be devoid of antibacterial activity, but extracts relax smooth muscle and have antipyretic activity, as well as antitumor activity in animals. This species has been shown to be devoid of alkaloids. Other species of *Celosia* that are used as herbal remedies outside of China are as follows: *C.leptostachys* for rheumatism, *C.stuhlmanniana* as an anthelmintic, and *C. cristata* as a diuretic. Experimentally, *C.coromandeliana* shows activity on the CNS and antipyretic activity, as well as antitumor and antiviral activity.

Activity Rating = +4,0

See activities listed for *Equisetum hiemale*.

*Cyathula capitata

Dried root

a. For rheumatoid arthritis, combine with Viscum coloratum, Gentiana macrophylla, Clematis chinensis, and then decoct.
b. For rheumatic fever, eczema and erysipelas, combine with Phellodendron amurense, Atractylodes lancea, and then decoct or grind to a powder.
c. For amenorrhea, combine with Angelica sinensis, Carthamus tinctorius, and then decoct.

A number of steroidal ecdysones have been isolated from this plant that could well be expected to elicit an anti-inflammatory response, although this type of activity has not yet been reported for this class of compounds. Ecdysterone, inokosterone, and cyasterone, all isolated from C.capitata, have been shown to stimulate protein synthesis in mouse liver preparations. The alkaloid gentianine is also known to have anti-inflammatory activity in laboratory animals and has been isolated from Gentiana macrophylla.
Viscum coloratum also would be expected to contribute to the antirheumatic effect of the prescription (a), since related Viscum species contain anti-inflammatory triterpenes. Several Clematis species have a folkloric reputation as being useful in the treatment of arthritis.

Activity Rating = +5,+5,0

APOCYNACEAE

√ Rauvolfia verticillata Dried root Activity Rating = +5,0	a. For hypertension, decoct alone. b. For furunculosis and snake bite.	Rauvolfia verticillata is a known source of the antihypertensive alkaloid reserpine, and is therefore justified as a Chinese Traditional medicine for the treatment of hypertension.

ARACEAE

√*_Acorus gramineus_
(_A. pseudoacorus_)
(Syn. _Acorus pseudoacorus_)

Dried rhizome

a. For sputum stuck in the throat, unconsciousness, deafness, chest congestion, and excessive dreams, decoct with _Poria cocos_, _Arisaema consanguineum_, _Citrus_ spp. and _Polygala tenuifolia_.
b. For chest and abdomen congestion or pain, anorexia, decoct with _Evodia rutaecarpa_, _Cyperus rotundus_, or decoct with _Magnolia officinalis_ and _Citrus_ spp.
c. For endless diarrhea, decoct with _Codonopsis pilosula_, _Nelumbo nucifera_ and _Poria cocos_.

Acorus gramineus has been shown to have antiviral activity, which is due to the volatile oil. The related _A. calamus_ has been shown to have piscicidal activity, relaxes smooth muscle, has insecticidal, antifungal, antibacterial, CNS depressant, hypotensive and hallucinogenic activity, affects respiration in rat brain, and has anticonvulsant activity. These activities are due mainly to alpha and beta asarones, which have the following pharmacologic effects: CNS depressant, anticonvulsant, and hypothermic.

The sesquiterpene acoric acid, from _A.calamus_, has anticonvulsant activity also. These asarones are also present in _A.gramineus_, thus this plant should also have the previously mentioned activities described for _A.calamus_. _Acorus calamus_ has also been used as an herbal remedy for the following: analgesic, hypotensive, sedative, anti-convulsant, anticancer, stomach disorders, aphrodisiac, female contraceptive, antipyretic, insecticide, anti-diarrheal, anthelmintic, anti-rheumatic, antibacterial, and as an anti-emetic.

Activity Rating = +5,+5,0

√ _Arisaema consanguineum_

Dried tubers

a. For cough with expectoration, combine with _Pinellia ternata_, _Atractylodes macrocephala_, and

The only work found concerned with _A.consanguineum_ was a report that it does not contain flavonoids, saponins

	Citrus spp., and then decoct. b. For coughs with expectoration and fever, combine with Pinellia ternata, Citrus spp., Atractylodes macrocephala and Scutellaria baicalensis, and then decoct. c. For dizziness, epilepsy, clonus, apoplexy and tetanus, combine with Pinellia ternata, Typhonium giganteum and Ledebouriella seseloides, and then decoct. d. For inflammation and snakebite, grind with vinegar and use externally.	or alkaloids. Other Arisaema species have shown anticancer activity in animals. Folkloric uses of other Arisaema species outside of China include: antifertility, antipyretic, analgesic, diuretic, anti-inflammatory, antifungal and anticancer. See pharmacological activities of Pinellia ternata (sedative, analgesic) and Scutellaria baicalensis (sedative).
Activity Rating = +5,+5,+5,0		
Pinellia ternata (Syn. Pinellia tuberifera) Dried tuber.	a. For use as an antitussive and expectorant, decoct with Citrus spp., Glycyrrhiza uralensis and Poria cocos. b. For pregnant vomiting or vomiting (stomach pain or intoxication), decoct with Perilla frutescens and Zingiber officinale. If fever is present, add Coptis chinensis. c. For chest pain, decoct with Coptis chinensis and Trichosanthes kirilowii.	Pinellia ternata has been used as a folkloric anticancer remedy, and this activity has been confirmed in animals. Extracts of this plant have shown analgesic activity in animals, as well as antiemetic and sedative activity, and the active principle is stated to be an uncharacterized sterol. See Coptis chinensis (analgesic).
Activity Rating = +5,+5,+5		
Typhonium giganteum Dried root.	a. Use alone as an anticonvulsant. b. For headache, apoplectic stroke, paralytic stroke or tetanus, decoct with Pinellia ternata, Arisaema consanguineum and Buthus martensi.	Typhonium giganteum has been used as a folkloric antidiabetic remedy. See Pinellia ternata (analgesic)
Activity Rating = 0,+5		

ARALIACEAE

Acanthopanax gracilistylus Dried root bark. Activity Rating = +5,0,0	a. For joint pain and convulsions of the limbs, prepare a tincture and take alone, or decoct with Angelica pubescens, Clematis chinensis, Morus alba and Spatholobus suberectus. b. For pediatric rickets, decoct or grind with Achyranthes bidentata and Chaenomeles lagenaria. c. For dysuria, dropsy and eczema and itching of the scrotum.	Nothing was found in the literature relative to the pharmacologic effects of Acanthopanax gracilistylus. However, extracts of A.sessiliflorum have been shown to increase non-specific resistance; extracts of A.sieboldiana elicit antiprogestational activity; and extracts of A.spinosus decreased conditioned avoidance responses in rats. See Angelica pubescens (anti-inflammatory)
Panax ginseng Dried root Activity Rating = 0,0,0	a. For weakness after vomiting of blood, for menorrhagia and for vomiting, decoct or use as a powder orally, or combine with Aconitum carmichaeli and then decoct. b. For rectocele, combine with Astragalus membranaceus and decoct. c. For fever, gasping, excessive sweating and thirst, combine with Ophiopogon japonicus and Schisandra chinensis and decoct.	None of the many pharmacological activities reported in over 500 original literature reports on Panax ginseng would account for the uses stated for this plant in Traditional Chinese medicine.
Tetrapanax papyriferum Dried stem pith Activity Rating = +3,+3,0,0	a. Alone, for water retention, diuretic, fever, and failure of lactation. b. As a diuretic, decoct with Poria cocos, talc, Alisma plantago-aquatica and Atractylodes macrocephala. c. For absence of lactation after labor, use alone cooked with hog's feet, or decoct with Vaccaria pyramidata, or decoct with Vaccaria pyramidata and Astragalus membranaceus.	Tetrapanax papyriferum has been used as a folkloric choleretic and diuretic. Experimentally, extracts of this plant have shown anticancer activity in laboratory animals.

ARISTOLOCHIACEAE

Aristolochia debilis Dried root and dried ripe fruit. Activity Rating = +5	a. Used the same as *Aristolochia contorta*.	See *Aristolochia contorta*.
Aristolochia contorta Dried ripe fruit Activity Rating = +5	a. For coughs with expectoration, combine with *Morus alba*, *Perilla frutescens*, *Arctium lappa* and *Glycyrrhiza uralensis*, and decoct.	There is nothing in the literature that would indicate that *A.contorta* should be useful as an expectorant. Other *Aristolochia* species have been used as herbal remedies outside of China for the following: anti-diarrheal, anthelmintic, analgesic, cardiotonic, diuretic, antipyretic, antibacterial, choleretic, fish poisoning, stomach ailments, female disorders, aphrodisiac, sedative, coughs, rheumatism, and antifertility. At least 20 species have been used for cancer remedies. In animals, aristolochic acid, which is present in most *Aristolochia* species, has been shown to be an active antitumor agent, but it is too toxic for clinical use. Other pharmacologic effects produced by various *Aristolochia* species are as follows: estrogenic, contraceptive, sedative, anticonvulsant, hallucinogenic, all determined in animals. Extracts have also shown *in vitro* antibacterial and antifungal activity. An alkaloid from *A.clematitis* has been shown to be a respiratory stimulant, to be diuretic, and act as a choleretic. See *Glycyrrhiza uralensis* (antitussive). See also *Aristolochia debilis* and *A.westlandi*.

Aristolochia westlandi Dried roots Activity Rating = +5,+3	a. For edema and beri-beri, combine with Astragalus membranaceus, Atractylodes macrocephala, Glycyrrhiza uralensis, and decoct. b. For aches, arthrodynia and numbness, combine with Clematis chinensis. Spatholobus suberectus, Bombyx mori, and then decoct.	See Aristolochia contorta and A.debilis. See Glycyrrhiza uralensis (diuretic).
Asarum heterotropoides var. mandshuricum Dried whole plant Activity Rating = 0,+5,0,0	a. For the common cold, headache, and stuffiness, combine with Schizonepeta tenuifolia, Ledebouriella seseloides, Ligusticum wallichii, and decoct. b. For chronic bronchitis and cough with expectoration, combine with Poria cocos, Glycyrrhiza uralensis, Schisandra chinensis, Zingiber officinale, and then decoct. c. For ulcers on the tongue and in the mouth, grind to a powder and apply topically. d. For nasal catarrh, combine with Ledebouriella seseloides and Angelica dahurica and decoct.	There is no information on this species. Asarum europaeum extracts injected into cats reduced or completely abolished neostigmine-induced bronchospasm. The flavonoids were found to be the active principles. Extracts of other Asarum species have shown the following effects: anticancer (the active principle is aristolochic acid), hormonal (due to beta sitosterol), CNS depressant, antiprotozoan, and in vitro antifungal, antibacterial and activities. See Glycyrrhiza uralensis (antitussive).
Hocquartia manshuriensis Dried root and stem. Activity Rating = 0,0,+4	a. Same uses as for Clematis montana.	Nothing was found in the literature with regard to the chemical constituents or pharmacological effects of H.manshuriensis.

ASCLEPIADACEAE

Cynanchum atratum Dried root Activity Rating = +4,+4,0	a. For fever and cough, combine with Artemisia apiacea, Lycium chinense, Rehmannia glutinosa, Eriobotrya japonica, and decoct. b. For hematuria and urethritis, combine with Paeonia lactiflora, Imperata cylindrica, and decoct. c. For anemia after parturition, combine with Angelica sinensis, Astragalus membranaceus, and decoct.	2-Hydroxy-4-methoxyacetophenone has been reported isolated from the related Cynanchum paniculatum, and has been shown to have antipyretic properties in rats with artificially induced fever. Related compounds, which presumably would have similar pharmacologic effects, have been isolated from several other Cynanchum species.
Cynanchum glaucescens Dried roots and stems Activity Rating = +5	Same uses as for Cynanchum stauntoni.	See Comments under C.atratum and C.stauntoni.
Cynanchum stauntoni Dried roots and stems Activity Rating = +5	a. For the common cold, cough, and irritated throat, combine with Aster tataricus, Glycyrrhiza uralensis, Perilla frutescens, Stemona sessilifolia, and decoct or grind to a powder. Take orally.	See comments under C.atratum above and see Glycyrrhiza uralensis (antitussive).
Periploca sepium Dried root bark. Activity Rating = +5	a. For gout, decoct with Clematis chinensis, Angelica pubescens and Morus alba.	All species of Periploca studied to date show cardiotonic effects and P.sepium has yielded the cardiac glycosides periplocin, periplocymarin, glycoside H-1, glycoside E, glycoside H and glycoside K. See Angelica pubescens (anti-inflammatory)

BERBERIDACEAE

Berberis amurensis

Dried roots and rhizomes.

a. For conjunctivitis, use as a decoction as an eye wash.
b. For furunculosis and inflammation, prepare a decoction and use orally as well as externally.

Berbamine, hydroxyberberine, jatrorrhizine and shobakumine have all been isolated from *Berberis amurensis* var. *japonica*, as well as berberine. Berberine has antibacterial properties, and has shown clinical efficacy as an antidiarrheal. Berberine is also active as an anticonvulsant, and has sedative activity as well as uterine stimulant activity. Berberine relaxes the smooth muscle of the intestine.

Activity Rating = +5,+5

BIGNONIACEAE

Campsis grandiflora

Dried flowers

a. For amenorrhea and dysmenorrhea, take the ground powder alone orally with wine, or decoct with _Angelica sinensis_, _Ligusticum wallichii_, _Carthamus tinctorius_ and the feces of _Trogopterus xanthipes_.
b. For urticaria and itching, take the ground powder orally with wine.
c. The root can be used for rheumatoid arthritis or monoplegia.

Nothing of value was found relative to _Campsis grandiflora_. _Campsis radicans_ extracts have been shown to exhibit insecticidal activity and CNS depressant activity.
Extracts of _Carthamus tinctorius_ relax smooth muscle.

Activity Rating = +5,0,0

BORAGINACEAE

√*Lithospermum erythrorhizon* Dried root	a. For eruptions, decoct with *Rehmannia glutinosa*, *Paeonia suffruticosa* and *Paeonia lactiflora*, or decoct with *Forsythia suspensa*, *Lonicera japonica* and *Glycyrrhiza uralensis*. b. For burns and eczema, decoct with sesame oil and use the oil externally, or decoct with *Rheum tanguticum*, *Angelica sinensis*, *Glycyrrhiza uralensis* and sesame oil and make an ointment for external application.	Nothing of value was found in the literature regarding *Lithospermum erythrorhizon* however *Lithospermum ruderale* has been used as a herbal remedy outside of China as a hemostatic, antidiarrheal, and as an oral contraceptive. Several *Lithospermum* species have shown antigonadotropic activity. *Lithospermum arvense* has been used as an herbal sedative, and as an oral contraceptive. Certain *Paeonia* species have shown antimicrobial activity *in vitro*, as well as *Forsythia suspensa* extracts. Certain *Angelica* species have also shown anti-inflammatory activity in animals, and *Glycyrrhiza uralensis* has anti-inflammatory triterpenes.
Activity Rating = +4,+5,+5,+5		
√ *Macrotomia euchroma* Dried roots	a. Used the same was as *Lithospermum erythrorhizon*.	Nothing of value was found relative to the chemical constituents or pharmacological activities of *Macrotomia euchroma*.
Activity Rating = 0		

CAMPANULACEAE

Codonopsis pilosula Dried root	a. For anorexia, combine with Atractylodes macrocephala, Poria cocos and Glycyrrhiza uralensis and decoct. b. For asthma, combine with Schisandra chinensis, Juglans sinensis and decoct. c. For weakness after a fever, combine with Ophiopogon japonicus and Schisandra chinensis and decoct. d. For insomnia, amnesia and palpitations, combine with Rehmannia glutinosa, Angelica sinensis and Polygala tenuifolia and decoct.	Codonopsis pilosula has been used as an herbal remedy for high blood pressure and for diabetes. A Russian species, Codonopsis lomonosovii, has been shown to increase the erythrocyte count in rabbits by 17.5 percent, as well as to increase the weight of the rabbits by 23 percent, when the extract was given orally. Rats showed a drop of 28-47 percent in urine excretion when administered this plant. The total glucosides from this plant prevented development of leucocytosis in rabbits after turpentine stimulus. See Angelica sinensis (sedative).
Activity Rating = +5,0,0,+5		
Lobelia chinensis Dried whole plant	a. For snake bite poisoning, decoct alone and take orally or triturate the fresh herb, drink the juice, and mix the marc with table salt and apply the mixture to the wound. Also can be used by preparing a decoction with Asarum heterotropoides var. mandshuricum, Scolopendra subspinipes mutilans, Buthus martensi and Prunella vulgaris. For edema, decoct alone.	No pharmacologic or chemical studies have been carried out on L.chinensis. The respiratory stimulant effect of most Lobelia species is well documented, and is due to the presence of lobeline and related alkaloids. Several species also contain the emetic alkaloid lobelanine and lobelanidine. However, data were not found that could explain the uses of L.chinensis in Chinese medicine.
Activity Rating = 0,0,0		
Platycodon grandiflorum Dried roots	a. For influenza, as an antitussive and expectorant, decoct with Schizonepeta tenuifolia, Cynanchum stauntoni and Glycyrrhiza uralensis.	An impure substance, designated as platycodin has been isolated from Platycodon grandiflorum and has been shown in animals to have analgesic,

b. For sore throat and tonsilitis, decoct with Lonicera japonica, Forsythia suspensa and Glycyrrhiza uralensis.

c. For lung pain and "sloughing ulcers", decoct with Taraxacum mongolicum, Amblytropis multiflora and Forsythia suspensa

sedative and antipyretic activity, as well as antihistaminic, anti-inflammatory and anticholinergic effects. It is also hypotensive and has expectorant properties, and completely inhibits gastric secretion in pylorus-ligated rats. Extracts of P.grandiflorum have also shown antitumor effects in animals (sloughing ulcer?). All of these effects (except the latter) have also been observed in humans by extracts of P.grandiflorum, thus confirming the value of this plant in Chinese medicine.

In prescription (a) Cynanchum stauntoni would be predicted to contain antipyretic substances.

In prescription (b) Lonicera japonica has been shown to exhibit in vitro antibacterial activity.

In prescription (c) Forsythia suspensa has been shown to exhibit antitumor properties in animals and may therefore explain its use for the treatment of "sloughing ulcers", which could be interpreted as being cancerous lesions.

Activity Rating = +5,+5,+5

CANNABACEAE

Cannabis sativa Dried ripe fruit	a. For constipation following fevers, decoct with *Prunus armeniaca*, *Thuja orientalis* and *Citrus aurantium*. b. For constipation following labor, decoct with *Thuja orientalis*, *Angelica sinensis* and *Rehmannia glutinosa*.	There is nothing in the literature concerning the chemical constituents or pharmacological activities of *Cannabis sativa* that would suggest that it would have laxative properties.

Activity Rating = 0,0

CAPPARIDACEAE

Gynandropsis gynandra

Dried ripe seed

a. For rheumatoid arthritis, decoct with water and use externally.
b. For bleeding hemorrhoids, decoct and use externally.
c. For malaria, use alone.

In Africa, G.gynandra is used as a native herbal remedy to reduce fever, for arthritis, for wound healing, as an anthelmintic, antibiotic, and analgesic. Extracts of this species have also been reported to have antitoxic properties.

Activity Rating = +3,+3,0

CAPRIFOLIACEAE

Lonicera japonica

Dried flowers

a. For fever and headache, decoct with Schizonepeta tenuifolia, Mentha arvensis, Glycyrrhiza uralensis.
b. For inflammations decoct with Chrysanthemum morifolium, Taraxacum mongolicum, Glycyrrhiza uralensis.
c. For diarrhea, decoct with Paeonia lactiflora, Glycyrrhiza uralensis, Saussurea lappa.
d. For arthritis, decoct with Morus alba.

No pharmacologic data have been found concerning any Lonicera species that would seem to support the uses attributed to L.japonica in Chinese medicine. However, an unspecified Lonicera species was alleged to be used widely in England for the treatment of gout, as a diuretic, for angina, to treat external ulcers, as an antispasmodic in asthma, and for coughs. However, L.japonica has been subjected to considerable pharmacological studies and extracts of this plant have been reported to have hypoglycemic as well as hyperglycemic activity, and to have antitumor, antibacterial, and antifungal activity.

See Glycyrrhiza uralensis (anti-inflammatory).

Activity Rating = +5,+5,0,0

CARYOPHYLLACEAE

Vaccaria pyramidata Dried ripe seed	a. For absence of lactation following labor, cook with one hog's foot and take orally. b. For mastitis and benign breast tumor, decoct with _Taraxacum mongolicum_, _Trichosanthes kirilowii_ and _Prunella vulgaris_. c. For amenorrhea, decoct with _Angelica sinensis_, _Ligusticum wallichii_, _Prunus persica_ and _Carthamus tinctorius_.	_Vaccaria pyramidata_ has been used as an herbal remedy for nephritis. Experimentally, extracts have shown _in vitro_ antibacterial effects. See _Taraxacum mongolicum_ (anticancer)

Activity Rating = 0,+5,0.

CHENOPODIACEAE

Kochia scoparia Dried ripe fruit Activity Rating = +5,+2	a. For skin infections, decoct alone and use orally or externally. b. For use as a diuretic, decoct with Grifola umbellata, Polygonum aviculare and Clematis montana.	Kochia scoparia is used as an herbal remedy in India as a cardiotonic agent (diuretic?). The plant is also considered to be toxic. Several unusual unsaturated fatty acids have been isolated from the seeds of K. scoparia, and these would be predicted to have antibacterial effects (skin infections?).
Salsola collina Dried whole plant Activity Rating = +5	a. For high blood pressure, decoct alone and take as a tea twice daily for six months.	Extracts of Salsola collina have been used clinically with success for the treatment of high blood pressure.

COMBRETACEAE

√ Quisqualis indica Dried ripe fruit or seed	a. For roundworm infestation, roast in a pan and take orally, or combine with Areca catechu and decoct. b. For "swelling of the belly", combine with Codonopsis pilosula, Atractylodes macrocephala and Glycyrrhiza uralensis and decoct. c. For worms in the bowels, decoct and take orally.	Quisqualis indica has been used as an herbal remedy outside of China as an anthelmintic. Experimentally, extracts of this plant have shown cathartic and antitumor activity in animals. See Areca catechu (anthelmintic).

Activity Rating = +3,+5,0,+3

COMMELINACEAE

<u>Commelina communis</u> Dried plant Activity Rating = 0,0,0	a. For fever, decoct and take orally. b. For mumps, obtain the juice from the plant and take orally, or combine with <u>Ajuga decumbens</u> and decoct. c. For bleeding, diarrhea and snake bite.	Extracts of <u>Commelina communis</u> show CNS depressant activity in mice, and antibacterial effects in human infections. The plant has been used as an herbal remedy for high blood pressure and as an antidiarrheal.

COMPOSITAE

*Arctium lappa Dried ripe fruit. Activity Rating = +5,+4,+5	a. For common cold and for sore throat, decoct with Lonicera japonica, Forsythia suspensa, Mentha arvensis and Glycyrrhiza uralensis. b. For erysipelas of the face and for epidemic parotitis, decoct with Schizonepeta tenuifolia, Ledebouriella seseloides, Cryptotympana atrata and Forsythia suspensa. c. For early symptoms of measles, huskiness of voice and for sore throat, decoct with Mentha arvensis, Cryptotympana atrata and Forsythia suspensa.	Arctium lappa has a long history of being used as a folkloric antibacterial remedy outside of China, as well as an anti-inflammatory, antipyretic, diuretic, and as a drug to "induce lust". Experimentally, extracts of Arctium lappa have shown diuretic activity, antitumor activity, antifungal activity (due to polyacetylenes), estrogenic activity, hypoglycemic activity, an antibacterial activity. The antibacterial principle has been isolated and partially characterized as a lactone.
Artemisia apiacea Whole plant Activity Rating = 0,+4,0	a. For vertigo, combine with Nelumbo nucifera, talc, Glycyrrhiza uralensis, and Tetrapanax papyrifera and decoct. b. For malaria and epistaxis, take the juice expressed from the plant orally, or combine with Rehmannia glutinosa, Anemarrhena asphodeloides, Paeonia suffruticosa and decoct. c. For night sweating, combine with Ampelopsis japonica, Gentiana macrophylla and Lycium chinense and decoct.	Nothing of value was found concerning the chemical constituents or pharmacological activities of Artemisia apiacea. See Artemisia capillaris. See Paeonia suffruticosa (antipyretic).
Artemisia capillaris Dried young plant	a. For jaundice, (light) constipation, fever and oligouria, decoct with Gardenia jasminoides and Rheum tanguticum. b. For jaundice (dark) and cold limbs, decoct with Aconitum carmichaeli and	The volatile oil of Artemisia capillaris has been shown to exhibit antifungal activity, and the antifungal principle has been isolated and shown to be capillin (an aromatic acetylene).

	Zingiber officinale.	An ointment containing the essential oil has been clinically evaluated and found to be effective as an antifungal preparation. Capillin has also been shown to have antibacterial activity in vitro. See also Rheum tanguticum (cathartic).
Activity Rating = +5,0		
*Aster tataricus Dried root	a. For colds, and coughs with excessive sputum, decoct with Schizonepeta tenuifolia, Platycodon grandiflorum and Cynanchum stauntoni. b. For whooping cough, decoct with Tussilago farfara, Stemona sessilifolia and Schisandra chinensis. c. For coughs and hemoptysis, decoct with Schisandra chinensis, Anemarrhena asphodeloides and Ophiopogon japonicus.	Aster tataricus is reported to have been used as an herbal remedy outside of China for asthma and for coughs. In animal studies, Aster tataricus has shown antitumor activity. Several other Aster species have shown CNS depressant activity in animals, antitumor activity, antiprotozoan activity, and in vitro antibacterial, antifungal and antiviral activity. See Platycodon grandiflorum (antitussive), as well as Tussilago farfara (antitussive).
Activity Rating = +5,+5,0		
Atractylodes lancea Dried rhizome	a. For dyspepsia, combine with Magnolia officinalis, Citrus spp., and Glycyrrhiza uralensis and decoct. b. For eczema and edema, combine with Phellodendron amurense and Achyranthes bidentata and grind to a powder and take orally. c. For nyctalopia, cook with pork liver or lamb liver and take orally.	Atractylodes lancea is reported to have been used as an herbal remedy outside of China for nephritis, but no chemical or pharmacological data are available on this species. Other species of Atractylodes have shown in vitro antiviral activity and estrogenic activity in animals. Folkloric remedy uses of other Atractylodes species include anticancer, wound healing, hypotensive, urinary disorders and antidiabetic. See also Atractylodes macrocephala.
Activity Rating = 0,+5,0		

√ *Artemisia argyi*

Dried leaves

a. For menorrhagia and bleeding during pregnancy or after labor, decoct with *Angelica sinensis*, *Rehmannia glutinosa*, *Paeonia lactiflora* and *Ligusticum wallichii*.
b. For vomiting of blood, epistaxis and bloody stools
decoct with *Rehmannia glutinosa*, *Thuja orientalis* and *Nelumbo nucifera*, or decoct with *Sanguisorba officinalis*, *Sophora japonica* and *Thuja orientalis*.
c. For constant diarrhea, decoct with *Zingiber officinalis* and *Citrus* spp.

Artemisia capillaris has been reported to have antibacterial and antifungal activity. The antifungal constituent has been isolated and identified as the aromatic acetylene capillin. Certain *Angelica* species have shown hemostatic properties in animals and *Sophora subprostrata* has shown anti-ulcer properties in animals.

Activity Rating = +4,0,0,+4,0

Atractylodes macrocephala Dried rhizome	a. As an aperient and for anorexia, combine with Codonopsis pilosula, Poria cocos and Glycyrrhiza uralensis and decoct, or combine with Codonopsis pilosula, Poria cocos, Dioscorea batatas and Citrus spp. and grind to a powder and take orally. b. For dyspepsia and anorexia, combine with Citrus aurantium, and Citrus spp. and decoct or grind to a powder and take orally. c. For chronic bronchitis, coughs and for gasping, combine with Cinnamomum cassia, Glycyrrhiza uralensis and Poria cocos and decoct. d. For anemia of pregnancy, combine with Angelica sinensis, Paeonia lactiflora, Ligusticum wallichii and Scutellaria baicalensis and decoct.	Atractylodes macrocephala has been used as an herbal remedy for high blood pressure, for nephritis and for diabetes. Extracts of this species have shown in vitro antiviral activity. See also Atractylodes lancea. See Glycyrrhiza uralensis (antitussive).

Activity Rating = +4,+4,0,+5,0

Bidens bipinnata Whole plant	a. For rheumatism, decoct alone and take orally, or decoct with Clerodendrum trichotomum and take orally. b. For weakness and jaundice, decoct alone and take orally, or decoct with Zizyphus jujuba. c. For snake bite, use the fresh stem juice orally and apply the marc externally, or decoct with Lobelia chinensis and take orally. d. For internal hemorrhages and furunculosis, appendicitis, high blood pressure and infant's tabes mesentericus, decoct and take orally.	Extracts of Bidens bipinnata have shown anticancer activity in animals, and a mixture of Bidens bipinnata and Clerodendrum trichotomum has been evaluated for anti-inflammatory activity in animals. A mixture of crude alkaloids and total steroids from this plant mixture was shown to have anti-inflammatory activity in animals. Bidens frondosa and Bidens polylepis have shown anticancer activity in animals, whereas extracts of Bidens pilosa have shown hypotensive activity in animals.

Activity Rating = +5,0,0,0,0

√ _Carthamus tinctorius_ Dried flowers	a. For menoxenia and dysmennorhea, decoct with _Ligusticum wallichii_, _Angelica sinensis_, _Cyperus rotundus_ and _Corydalis bulbosa_, or prepare a tincture with _Angelica sinensis_ and take orally before the menstrual cycle. b. For amenorrhea, decoct with _Angelica sinensis_, _Prunus persica_ and _Sparganium stoloniferum_. c. For clots remaining after labor, and for abdominal pain, decoct with _Leonurus heterophyllus_, _Crataegus pinnatifida_ and black sugar. d. For internal hemorrhage and pain, decoct with _Bupleurum scorzonerae-folium_, _Angelica sinensis_, _Prunus persica_ and _Rheum tanguticum_ with wine and water.	_Carthamus tinctorius_ has been used outside of China as an herbal cathartic. Extracts of this plant have been shown to have cathartic activity and the active principles have been identified as 2-hydroxyactiin and matairesinol monoglucoside, two novel lignans. Extracts of _Carthamus tinctorius_ have also been shown to relax smooth muscle _in situ_, and to elicit antibacterial activity _in vitro_. See also _Angelica sinensis_ (smooth muscle relaxant) and _Leonurus heterophyllus_ (hemostatic).
Activity Rating = +5,0,+5,0		
√ _Centipeda minima_ Whole plant	a. For sinus congestion, grind to a powder and use externally. b. For whooping cough, decoct alone and take orally with honey. c. For snake bite, grind the fresh plant and use externally.	Extracts of _Centipeda minima_ have been shown to relax smooth muscle _in vitro_ and the plant has been used as an herbal remedy as an anticonvulsant. The following substances have been isolated from _Centipeda minima_: taraxasterol palmitate, taraxasterol acetate, taraxasterol, stigmasterol, beta sitosterol, arnidiol, lupeol acetate, lupeol, and hexacosanol.
Activity Rating = 0,+5,0		
√ _Cephalanoplsis segetum_ Dried whole plant	a. For hematuria, decoct with _Rehmannia glutinosa_, _Gardenia jasminoides_, _Typha latifolia_ and	Nothing of value was found concerning the chemical constituents or pharmacological activities of _Cephalanopsis_

	talc. b. For vomiting of blood, decoct with Gardenia jasminoides, Cirsium japonicum, Thuja orientalis and Agrimonia viscidula. c. For epidemic hepatitis and hepatomegaly, decoct the fresh root and take orally for ten days.	species of plants.
Activity Rating = 0,0,0		
Chrysanthemum indicum Dried flowers	a. For various skin infections, decoct alone (or decoct the fresh stem), or decoct with Taraxacum mongolicum, Lonicera japonica and Prunella vulgaris and take orally as well as use externally. b. For high blood pressure, use as a tea.	**Chrysanthemum indicum has been used as an herbal antibiotic outside of China, as well as for high blood pressure. Extracts of this plant have shown insect moulting activity.**
Activity Rating = +5,+3		
Chrysanthemum morifolium Dried flowers	a. For the common cold, combine with Morus alba, Prunus armeniaca, Mentha arvensis and Phragmites communis and decoct. b. For headache, combine with Prunella vulgaris, Lamprotula leai, Bombyx mori and Uncaria rhynchophylla and decoct. c. For conjunctivitis, combine with Equisetum hiemale, Cryptotympana atrata and Tribulus terrestris and decoct. d. For dizziness, vertigo and xerosis conjunctivae, combine with Rehmannia glutinosa and Lycium chinense and decoct.	Chrysanthemum morifolium has been reported to produce an irritant effect in humans, and the principle responsible for this is probably the sesquiterpene lactone chlorochrymorin. See also Chrysanthemum indicum. See Equisetum hiemale (antibacterial).
Activity Rating = 0,0,+5,0		

Cirsium japonicum Dried whole plant	a. For hemoptysis and vomiting of blood, take the juice of the plant orally, or combine with Nelumbo nucifera, Thuja orientalis, Imperata cylindrica and Rubia cordifolia, roast in a pan, grind to a powder and take orally. b. For epistaxis, combine with Thuja orientalis, Nelumbo nucifera, Artemisia argyi and Selaginella tamarascina and decoct. c. For metrorrhagia, combine with Nelumbo nucifera, Zizyphus jujuba and Typha latifolia and decoct. d. For hematuria, take the juice from the plant orally. e. For inflammations, take the juice of the plant orally or use externally.	Nothing was found concerning the chemical constituents or pharmacological activities of Cirsium japonicum that would explain the use of this plant in Traditional Chinese medicine.

Activity Rating = 0,0,0,0,0,0

Eclipta prostrata (Syn. Eclipta alba, E.punctata). Dried whole plant	a. For dizziness, vomiting of blood and lumbago, combine with Ligustrum lucidum, grind to a powder and take orally, or combine with Ligustrum lucidum and Morus alba and decoct. b. For enterorrhagia, and bleeding in the lungs, decoct and take orally, or combine with Thuja orientalis, Agrimonia viscidula and Sanguisorba officinalis and decoct. c. For hematuria, combine with Plantago asiatica, squeeze out the juice, and take orally. d. For copremia, decoct and take orally. e. For bleeding from cuts, grind to a powder and use externally.	Eclipta prostrata has been used as an herbal remedy outside of China as a hemostatic, for cancer, as a tonic, a deobstruant, for hepatic and splenic enlargement, and for scorpion stings as well as for stomach ailments, for high blood pressure, as a choleretic, analegesic, diuretic, for fevers, and for rheumatism. Experimentally, extracts of this plant show estrogenic activity (due to norwedelolactone), cardiovascular effects, relax smooth muscle and have insecticide activity.

Activity Rating = 0,0,+5,0,0,+3

*Eupatorium fortunei Dried whole plant	a. For anorexia, add water to fresh leaves or decoct dried whole plant with Atractylodes lancea, Agastache rugosa, Citrus spp. and Nelumbo nucifera.	Nothing can be said with regard to the justification of this use based on pharmacological reports on this or related Eupatorium species.
Activity Rating = 0		
Gynura segetum Dried roots	a. For contusions, decoct with water and wine and use externally. b. For snake bite, furunculosis and bleeding, use alone.	No information of value was found in the literature regarding this genus of plant.
Activity Rating = 0,0		
Inula japonica Dried flower heads	a. For cough, excess sputum and chest congestion, decoct with Prunus armeniaca, Morus alba and Perilla frutescens. b. For cough, gasping, fevers and chills (alternating), decoct with Schizonepeta tenuifolia, Peucedanum praeruptorum, Pinellia ternata and Asarum heterotropoides. c. For spleen and stomach ailments, chills and chest congestion, decoct with Pinellia ternata, Codonopsis pilosula and Zingiber officinale.	Some novel sesquiterpene lactones have been isolated from Inula japonica, and compounds of this type are known to have antimicrobial activity. A related species, Inula grantioides, has been reported to be useful as an anti-asthmatic. See Asarum heterotropoides (antitussive).
Activity Rating = +5,+5,0		
Saussurea lappa Dried root	a. For dyspepsia, decoct with Codonopsis pilosula, Atractylodes macrocephala, Pinellia ternata and Citrus spp. b. For gas and tympanites of the abdomen, decoct with Atractylodes macrocephala and Citrus aurantium. c. For dysentery and abdominal	Saussurea lappa has a broad reputation as being useful for such conditions as stomach disorders, and as tonics, bitters, antiseptics, antidiarrheals, antiviral agents, aphrodisiacs, contraceptives, and for female disorders, as well as to lower blood cholesterol levels. On the experimental side,

	pain, decoct or grind with *Coptis chinensis* and take orally.	extracts of this plant have been evaluated in animals and have been shown to have antispasmodic and hypertensive, antitumor and insecticide activity, but are devoid of antibacterial activity. The essential oil from this plant shows *in vitro* antiviral activity. Extracts of *Saussurea lappa* have been subjected to general pharmacological screening, but details of these studies were not immediately available. The pharmacological activity appears to reside in an uncharacterized alkaloid fraction. See *Coptis chinensis* (antidiarrheal).
Activity Rating = 0,0,+5		
✓ *Siegesbeckia pubescens* Dried whole plant	a. For rheumatoid arthritis, convulsions and paralytic stroke, grind the drug and take orally by itself, or grind with *Clerodendrum trichotomum*, *Acanthopanax gracilistylis* (or *Periploca sepium*) and *Xanthium strumarium*.	No literature reports have been found that would substantiate the uses for *Siegesbeckia pubescens* in Chinese medicine. Extracts of *Clerodendrum trichotomum* have shown anti-inflammatory activity in animals.
Activity Rating = 0,+5		
✓ *Sonchus brachyotus* Dried whole plant	a. For appendicitis, decoct with rice (*Oryza sativa*) and *Aconitum carmichaeli*. b. For dermatitis and inflammation, decoct alone or with *Amblytropis multiflora*. c. For vaginal discharges and abdominal pain, including that from after labor, decoct alone and take orally.	Nothing of value concerning the chemical constituents or pharmacological effects of *Sonchus brachyotus* was found in the literature. See *Aconitum carmichaeli* (antibacterial activity).
Activity Rating = +5,0,0		

Taraxacum mongolicum Dried whole plant with roots.	a. Decoct alone for fever and inflammation. b. For mastitis, decoct alone for use or decoct with Trichosanthes kirilowii, Forsythia suspensa and Angelica dahurica. c. For dermatitis inflammation, decoct with Chrysanthemum morifolium, Lonicera japonica and Glycyrrhiza uralensis. d. For acute hepatitis, decoct with Artemisia capillaris, Fraxinus rhynchophylla and Rheum tanguticum. e. For appendicitis, decoct with Amblytropis multiflora, Portulaca oleracea, Scutellaria baicalensis and Salvia miltiorhiza.	No data could be found concerning Taraxacum mongolicum. However, Taraxacum officinale extracts have been reported to have the following activities in laboratory animals: diuretic, hypoglycemic, antispasmodic (due to a flavonoid glycoside), anticancer, choleretic, and in vitro, antibacterial, and antifungal activities. See Glycyrrhiza uralensis (anti-inflammatory).
Activity Rating = 0,+5,+5,0,+5		
Tussilago farfara Dried flower buds	a. Use alone as an antitussive. b. For chronic cough and bronchitis, decoct with Aster tataricus and Anemarrhena asphodeloides, or triturate with Lilium brownii and honey.	Tussilago farfara has been used as a herbal remedy for asthma, as an antitussive, and as an antibacterial. Experimentally, extracts have shown CNS depressant in vitro antibacterial and antitussive activity. Pectins have been isolated from the leaves of Tussilago farfara, and this could, in part, account for its used in Traditional Chinese medicine for the treatment of coughs, due to the soothing and demulcent effects known to be produced by pectins.
Activity Rating = +5,+5,+5		
Xanthium strumarium Dried ripe fruit	a. For the common cold and headache, combine with Angelica dahurica and Perilla frutescens, and decoct. b. For rheumatic pain and arthritis, combine with Phellodendron amurense	The total alkaloids of Xanthium strumarium have been shown to elicit a respiratory stimulant effect in rabbits, as well as to relax the smooth muscle of the small intestine.

and Atractylodes lancea and decoct.
c. For rhinitis, combine with Ligusticum wallichii, Angelica dahurica and Mentha arvensis and decoct.
d. External use for eczema and rubella, decoct the stems and leaves with water and apply externally.

Extracts of this species also show antitumor properties in laboratory animals, and elicit a hypoglycemic effect. Carveol has been isolated from this plant, and it has been shown to have CNS stimulant properties in animals.

Activity Rating = 0,0,+5,0

CONVOLVULACEAE

Cuscuta chinensis Dried ripe seed Activity Rating = 0,0,+3,+5	a. For notalgia, lumbago, emissions, hypogonadism, enuresis and polyuria, combine with Rosa laevigata, Hierodula sp., and Schisandra chinensis, and then decoct. b. For dizziness, combine with Rehmannia glutinosa, and Plantago asiatica, and then decoct. c. For "weakness in pregnancy" or for miscarriages, combine with Viscum coloratum and Dipsacus asper, and then decoct. d. For weakness, combine with Codonopsis pilosula, Dioscorea batatas, Lycium chinensis, and Nelumbo nucifera, and then decoct.	Cuscuta chinensis is reported useful as a diuretic and to treat female disorders in other countries.
*Ipomoea hederacea Dried ripe seed Activity Rating = 0,+5	a. For edema, anuria and constipation, grind the seeds and take orally. b. For ascariasis, grind the seeds with Areca catechu and Rehmannia glutinosa and take orally.	Very little has been published concerning I.hederacea. However, many Ipomoea species are known to contain very active cathartic glycoresins, but these are found only in the tubers and not in the seeds. The seeds of I. hederacea are reported to contain lysergol, chanoclavine, penniclavine, isopenniclavine and elymoclavine, but the known pharmacological activities of these indole alkaloids cannot account for the medicinal effects attributed to I.hederacea in Chinese medicine. Ipomoea hederacea seeds are reported to be hallucinogenic when ingested by humans. The prescription containing I.hederacea, Areca catechu and Rehmannia glutinosa, would undoubtedly be effective in ascariasis, since A.catechu contains the known anthelmintic arecoline.

CORNACEAE

Cornus officinalis

Dried fruit without seeds

a. For lumbago and dizziness, combine with *Rehmannia glutinosa*, *Dioscorea batatas*, *Poria cocos* (a fungus), *Alisma plantago-aquatica*, and then decoct.
b. For polyuria, combine with *Hierodula* sp. and *Dioscorea batatas*, and then decoct.
c. For "emissions", combine with *Rosa laevigata*, *Ligustrum lucidum*, and then decoct.
d. For night sweating, combine with *Schisandra chinensis*, *Codonopsis pilosula*, *Ostrea* sp., *Astragalus membranaceus*, and then decoct.

A quinol glucoside has been isolated from *C. officinalis*, which could be expected to act as a urinary antiseptic, and this could be the reason for the alleged effectiveness of this plant in treating polyuria. Extracts of *C. officinalis* have been shown to elicit antibacterial activity against *Staphylococcus aureus in vitro*, *Salmonella typhosa* and *Shigella dysenteriae*.
Aqueous and alcoholic extracts of *C. officinalis* fruits have elicited antiallergenic effects as shown by measurement of the amount of anaphylactic mediator released from the chopped tissue of sensitized guinea pig lung challenged with the specific antigen. The mediator was decreased by 20-40 per cent.
In prescription (a), *Dioscorea batatas* would be expected to contain diosgenin, which has been shown to exhibit anti-inflammatory activity in animals.

Activity Rating = +5,0,0,0

CRUCIFERAE

Capsella bursa-pastoris

Whole plant

a. For dysentery and diarrhea, decoct alone and take orally or decoct with *Pteris multifida*.
b. For chyluria and menorrhagia, decoct the fresh plant and take orally.
c. For tuberculosis of the kidney, cook the dry plant with egg and take orally.
d. For ophthalmia, hypertension and hemorrhages, decoct and take orally.

Capsella bursa-pastoris has been used as an herbal remedy outside of China for the treatment of cancer, as a bitter, diuretic, antidiarrheal and for arthritis, as a contraceptive and as an antipyretic. Experimentally, this species has shown hypotensive activity, anticancer activity, cardiotonic, vasodilator, smooth muscle relaxant, sedative, hormonal and antifertility activity. Extracts of this plant also have uterine stimulant activity and produce effects on the central nervous system. The uterine stimulant principles have been isolated, but have not as yet been characterized. The presence of isothiocyanates in this plant would explain its antimicrobial effects.

Activity Rating = +3,+5,+5,+5

Descurainia sophia

Dried ripe seeds

a. For cough, gasping, and excess sputum, decoct with the date, *Prunus armeniaca* and *Ephedra sinica*.
b. For edema, and dysuria, decoct with *Aristolochia westlandi* and *Rheum tanguticum*.

Nothing was found in the literature regarding the pharmacological effects of *Descurainia* species. The ephedrine present in *Ephedra sinica* is responsible for the antitussive effect and the *Prunus armeniaca* (dates) are undoubtedly contributing a demulcent effect due to the high concentrations of mucilage and sugars.

Activity Rating = +5,+4

Isatis tinctoria Dried roots and leaves	a. For acute fever, sore throat and rash, decoct alone or with Rehmannia glutinosa, Scrophularia ningpoensis and Glycyrrhiza uralensis. b. For parotitis, decoct alone and use orally or externally, or decoct with Forsythia suspensa, Arctium lappa and Scutellaria baicalensis.	An 80 per cent acetone extract of the roots of I.tinctoria has been reported to be active against both Gram positive and Gram negative organisms, which explains most of the medicinal applications of this plant. Further, Forsythia suspensa would be expected to contain antipyretic and analgesic constituents (see Forsythia suspensa). It also has antibacterial properties.
Activity Rating = +5,+5		
Lepidium apetalum Dried roots	a. For the common cold and for cough, decoct with Mentha arvensis, Arctium lappa, Prunus armeniaca and Platycodon grandiflorum. b. For choking of the chest and for excess sputum, decoct with Perilla frutescens, Citrus sp. and Citrus aurantium.	Lepidium apetalum has not been reported to be pharmacologically or chemically investigated. However, it is apparent that isothiocyanate compounds are ubiquitous in members of this genus, and these compounds are known to have antibacterial activity. Further, Lepidium species are rich in mucilages, which could contribute to their application as cough remedies. Several Lepidium species have been reported to elicit hypotensive activity and to relax smooth muscle. In prescription (a) Platycodon grandiflorum has been shown to contain platycodin, a substance having antitussive properties.
Activity Rating = +5,0		
Raphanus sativus Seed, leaf and old root.	a. For diarrhea, and tympanites of the abdomen, decoct with Crataegus pinnatifida (or Crataegus cuneata),	Raphanus sativus has been used as an herbal remedy for arthritis, cancer, as a diuretic, for nephritis, and for

or pulverize into a powder.

b. For use as an antitussive and antiasthmatic, decoct with the seed of Perilla frutescens.

c. For dysentery and diarrhea, decoct alone and take orally.

d. For edema, malnutrition, tympanites of the abdomen, and oligouria, decoct the root with Poria cocos, Atractylodes macrocephala and Citrus spp.

female disorders. Experimentally, the antitumor activity has been confirmed, as well as the diuretic effects. Extracts of this plant have shown in vitro antibacterial, antifungal, and antiviral effects. The active antibacterial and antifungal principle has been identified as raphanin.

See Crataegus pinnatifida (antidiarrheal).

Activity Rating = +5,0,+5,+3

CUCURBITACEAE

Trichosanthes kirilowii Dried fruit, seed and root	a. For use as an expectorant, use alone or decoct with Platycodon grandiflorum and Prunus armeniaca. b. For mastitis, decoct with Lonicera japonica and Taraxacum mongolicum. c. For chest congestion and discomfort, decoct with Coptis chinensis and Pinellia ternata. d. For constipation, use a decoction of the seed. e. For fever, thirst, anxiety and inflammation, decoct with Scrophularia ningpoensis, Lonicera japonica and Glycyrrhiza uralensis. f. For diabetes, decoct with Dioscorea batatas, Anemarrhena asphodeloides and Cornus officinalis.	Trichosanthes kirilowii has been reported to be devoid of hypoglycemic effects in normal as well as alloxan-treated rabbits, but other investigators have reported that extracts of this plant produce hypoglycemia in laboratory animals. This species has been used outside of China as a folkloric remedy to treat infections. In prescription (a) Platycodon grandiflorum contains platycodin, a substance shown to have expectorant properties. In prescription (d), most plants in the Cucurbitaceae family contain unusual triterpenes (cucurbitacins), which are known to have cathartic properties. In prescription (e) Glycyrrhiza uralensis is known to contain several flavonoids and glycyrrhizin, all of which show anti-inflammatory activity in animals.
Activity Rating = +5,0,0,+5,+5		
Trichosanthes multiloba Fruit and seed	a. For the same conditions as Trichosanthes kirilowii.	See comments under Trichosanthes kirilowii.
Activity Rating = +5,0,0,+5,+4		

CUPRESSACEAE

Thuja orientalis Dried ripe seed, leaves and twigs	a. Use alone as a decoction as a sedative, for minor headaches, and as a coagulant. Decoct the seeds with Angelica sinensis, Rehmannia glutinosa, Polygonum multiflorum and Ostrea spp. b. For constipation, decoct with Cannabis sativa. c. For bleeding of the nostrils and vomiting of blood, decoct the leaf with Rehmannia glutinosa, Scrophularia ningpoensis, Nelumbo nucifera and Imperata cylindrica. d. For bloody urine, decoct the leaf with Cephalanopsis segetum and Imperata cylindrica. e. For bloody feces (hemorrhoids?), decoct with Sophora japonica, Schizonepeta tenuifolia and Citrus aurantium. f. For early menses and menorrhagia, decoct with Rehmannia glutinosa, Rubia cordifolia, Ligusticum lucidum and Nelumbo nucifera.	Thuja orientalis has been used as an herbal remedy for cancer and lignans that would be predicted to have antitumor activity are widespread in the genus Thuja, although none have specifically been isolated from Thuja orientalis.

Activity Rating = +5,0,0,0,0,0

CYPERACEAE

Cyperus rotundus Dried tuber	a. For menoxenia and dysmenorrhea, combine with Angelica sinensis, Paeonia lactiflora, Ligusticum wallichii, Artemisia argyi, and Cocculus laurifolius, and decoct. b. For chest pains, combine with Citrus aurantium, Paeonia lactiflora, Glycyrrhiza uralensis and decoct. c. For stomach ache, combine with Zingiber officinale, Saussurea lappa and Pinellia ternata and then decoct.	Cyperus rotundus has been used as an herbal remedy for pain, cancer, and for high blood pressure. An essential oil from this plant has shown in vitro antibacterial effects against Gram positive organisms; an extract of the roots inhibited 14 fungi in vitro, and the volatile oil has shown in vitro antiviral activity. Alcoholic and aqueous extracts have been reported to stimulate the frog heart in situ, and gave a prolonged hypotensive and vasodilating effect. Similar extracts showed a diuretic effect, tranquilizing activity, relaxed smooth muscle, acted as an antiemetic, showed antipyretic, anti-inflammatory, hypotensive, antihistaminic and analgesic activity.

Activity Rating = +5,+5,+5

DIOSCOREACEAE

Dioscorea batatas Dried tuber	a. For weakness and diarrhea, combine with Codonopsis pilosula and Atractylodes macrocephala and decoct. b. For coughs, premature ejaculations, enuresis and polyuria, combine with Rehmannia glutinosa, Cornus officinalis and Schisandra chinensis and decoct. c. For leucorrhea, combine with Atractylodes macrocephala, Plantago asiatica, Sepia esculenta and Rubia cordifolia and decoct. d. For polyuria, combine with Ophiopogon japonicus, Trichosanthes kirilowii and Anemarrhena asphodeloides and decoct.	No information was found concerning the pharmacological activities of chemical constituents of Dioscorea batatas. Dioscorea bulbifera has shown anticancer activity in animals, as has Dioscorea villosa. Dioscorea oppositifolia has shown anti-inflammatory activity, undoubtedly due to the steroidal saponins, as well as antidiarrheal effects. Several Dioscorea species have shown in vitro antifungal activity, and a saponin of unknown structure from an unspecified Dioscorea species has been shown to lower blood cholesterol levels in animals. Dioscorea batatas has been shown to contain considerable amounts of mucilage, which could explain its use as a cough remedy, due to an emollient and soothing effect on mucous membranes.
Activity Rating = +5,+5,0,+5		
Dioscorea nipponica Dried rhizomes	a. For rheumatoid arthritis, decoct alone or with black sugar, or macerate in wine for one week.	Diosgenin, a steroidal sapogenin, has been isolated from D.nipponica, and has been shown to elicit a 50 percent anti-inflammatory response against kaolin-induced rat paw edema when compared with suitable controls. Diosgenin is also an active anti-inflammatory agent in man. See also Dioscorea batatas.
Activity Rating = +5		

DIPSACACEAE

Dipsacus asper

Dried root

a. For weakness, lumbago, notalgia, combine with Viscum coloratum, Angelica sinensis, Cuscuta chinensis, and then decoct.
b. For trauma due to a fall, combine with Angelica sinensis, Corydalis bulbosa, Eupholyphaga sinensis, Ligusticum wallichii, and decoct.
c. For rheumatic pain, combine with Gentiana macrophylla, Morus alba, Cyathula capitata, Ledebouriella seseloides, and decoct.
d. For menorrhagia, combine with Rehmannia glutinosa, Angelica sinensis, Ligusticum wallichii, Artemisia argyi, and decoct.

Gentianine is an alkaloid known to be present in many Dipsacus species, although it has not been reported to date from D.asper. This alkaloid has been well documented by several groups to have anti-inflammatory activity in laboratory animals, and if present in D.asper, could account for the use of this plant in the treatment of arthritis. Dipsacus chinensis also has a folkloric reputation as being a useful treatment for arthritis outside of China.

Activity Rating = +4,+4,+5,+5

EPHEDRACEAE

√ *Ephedra sinica

Dried fresh branches and roots

a. For influenza, sweating and as an antitussive, decoct with Cinnamomum cassia, Glycyrrhiza uralensis and Prunus armeniaca.
b. For lung fever, asthma and as an antitussive, decoct with Prunus armeniaca, Glycyrrhiza uralensis and gypsum.
c. For chronic bronchitis, decoct ginger, Asarum heterotropoides and Pinellia ternata.
d. For edema and oligouria, decoct with Prunus armeniaca, Raphanus sativus and winter melon.
e. For night sweating, decoct with Ostrea sp. and wheat.

The use of Ephedra sinica for all of the conditions listed can be explained by the well-known presence of the alkaloid ephedrine in this species. Ephedrine is known to elicit all of these effects. The Cinnamomum cassia (cinnamon) is undoubtedly present to improve the taste of the prescription, and the Glycyrrhiza uralensis as a sweetening agent (it contains glycyrrhizin, which is 50 times sweeter than sugar, and also is responsible for the licorice taste). The Prunus armeniaca (dates) is probably present for its demulcent effects due to the presence of mucilage and high concentration of sugars.

See Glycyrrhiza uralensis (antitussive).

Activity Rating = +5,+5,+5,0,0

EQUISETACEAE

Equisetum hiemale

Dried whole plant

a. For ophthalmic conditions, decoct with *Morus alba*, *Chrysanthemum morifolium*, *Taraxacum mongolicum* and *Scutellaria baicalensis*.

b. For vertigo, pulverize with *Atractylodes lancea* and take with water.

c. For "cloudy eye", decoct with *Eriocaulon buergerianum*, *Cassia tora* and *Cryptotympana atrata*.

Equisetum hiemale contains several polyphenolic flavonoids which predictably would exert a mild antibacterial effect, thus perhaps substantiating the use of extracts of this plant for ophthalmic conditions (infections?)

Activity Rating = +5,0,+5

ERIOCAULACEAE

Eriocaulon buergerianum

Flower head with peduncle

a. For fever, headache, ophthalmia, or eye or tooth pain, decoct with *Gentiana scabra*, *Rehmannia glutinosa*, *Paeonia lactiflora* and *Carthamus tinctorius*.
b. For nyctalopia, cook with lamb or pork liver and eat the liver and soup.
c. For "cloudy eye", induced by *tabes mesentericus* (in children), decoct with *Cryptotympana atrata*, *Chrysanthemum morifolium* and *Equisetum hiemale*.

Nothing of value was found in the literature regarding the chemical constituents or pharmacological effects of members of the genus *Eriocaulon*.

Activity Rating = 0,0,+4

EUCOMMIACEAE

Eucommia ulmoides

Dried bark

a. For impotence, notalgia, lumbago, polyuria and leg and knee weakness, cook with pork kidney or decoct with Rehmannia glutinosa, Cuscuta chinensis, Dipsacus asper and walnut. (Juglans spp.)
b. For notalgia in pregnancy and lumbago, pulverize with Dipsacus asper and take with Zizyphus jujuba.
c. For initial stages of hypertension, decoct with water alone or with Prunella vulgaris and Scutellaria baicalensis.

Eucommia ulmoides infusions have been used in the treatment of hypertension in the USSR, with reported good results. Also, in the USSR, this effect has been confirmed in laboratory animals. In a paper published in 1956 from the Academia Sinica in Shanghai, it was concluded that although in hypertensive dog experiments a blood pressure drop was observed with extracts of E.ulmoides accompanied by a slowing of the heart rate, the overall effect was not great enough to warrant clinical use of E.ulmoides in the treatment of hypertension.
In prescription (a)and (b), anti-inflammatory activity is probably due to the alkaloid gentiamine, which is present in almost all Dipsacus species.

Activity Rating = +5,+5,+5

EUPHORBIACEAE

Acalypha australis Whole plant	a. For dysentery, diarrhea and enteritis, decoct alone or take as a ground powder orally. b. For vomiting of blood, decoct alone and take orally or decoct with Agrimonia viscidula. For pediatric tabes mesentericus, decoct alone and take orally or cook with hog liver. c. For different types of hemorrhages and eczema, decoct and take orally.	No information was found concerning Acalypha australis, however, several Acalypha species have been used as herbal remedies outside of China as follows: A.glomerata as an antiprotozoan, A.ornata for wound healing, A.sinensis for asthma and as an aphrodisiac, A.chirindica for nephritis, A.ciliata and A.indica as antitussives and antiemetics, A.septemloba, A.hederacea, A.hypogaea, A.phleoides and A.lindheimeri for treatment of cancer, and the latter species for the treatment of dysentery. Experimentally, A.lanceolata and A.phleoides have shown anticancer activity in animals, A.virginiana has shown antibacterial but not antifungal activity in vitro, and A.balfourii has shown in vitro antibacterial activity.
Activity Rating = +2,0,+4		
*Euphorbia humifusa Dried whole plant	a. For dysentery, decoct alone or with Acalypha australis. b. For prolonged bleeding, take the powdered plant with wine.	Nothing of interest has been found on the pharmacology of Euphorbia humifusa. See Acalypha australis (antidiarrheal).
Activity Rating = +5,+2		
*Euphorbia kansui Dried roots	a. For ascites, dysuria and constipation, decoct with Ipomoea hederacea and Zizyphus jujuba. b. For hydrothorax, use alone.	Recently toxic (irritant) diterpene esters have been isolated from Euphorbia kansui, which could explain the laxative effect.
Activity Rating = +5,0		

GENTIANACEAE

Gentiana macrophylla

Dried roots

a. For rheumatoid arthritis, decoct alone or combine with Angelica pubescens, Viscum coloratum, Clematis chinensis and decoct.
b. For fever, combine with Anemarrhena asphodeloides, Lycium chinensis, Artemisia apiacea and decoct.
c. For jaundice and hemorrhoids, decoct alone.

Virtually every species of Gentiana studied to date has yielded the alkaloid gentianine. This alkaloid has been reported by several different investigators to have anti-inflammatory activity in laboratory animals. Gentianine has been isolated from G. macrophylla, thus this species, used in Chinese medicine for the treatment of rheumatoid arthritis, has a rational basis for this action. Extracts of G.macrophylla have not been reported to act on the liver directly, but extracts of the related G.lutea have been shown to exhibit a choleretic effect in laboratory animals.

See also Gentiana scabra.

Activity Rating = +5,0,+4

Gentiana scabra

Dried roots

a. For inflammations of the eye, combine with Bupleurum scorzonerae-folium, Gardenia jasminoides, Scutellaria baicalensis and Plantago asiatica, and decoct.
b. For rheumatoid arthritis and jaundice, decoct with Gardenia jasminoides and Sophora flavescens.
c. For fevers and the common cold, combine with Bombyx mori, Uncaria rhynchophylla and Coptis chinensis and prepare a decoction.

The use of G.scabra for inflammatory conditions seems logical on the basis that the known anti-inflammatory alkaloid gentianine should be present in this species. Two other species of Gentiana have been shown to elicit antibacterial activity in vitro

See also Gentiana macrophylla.

Activity Rating = +5,+5,0

GINKGOACEAE		
Ginkgo biloba Dried ripe seed	a. For asthma and cough with expectoration, decoct with Ephedra sinica and Glycyrrhiza uralensis. b. For leucorrhea, combine with Nelumbo nucifera, Sepia esculenta and decoct. c. For tuberculosis, decoct alone.	The biflavonoid fraction from G. biloba has been shown to relax smooth muscle (asthma?), as well as to have antibradykinin activity in guinea pig ileum. The sesquiterpene lactone, bilobalide, and the diterpene lactone ginkgolide A, both isolated from G.biloba, have been shown to have antibacterial activity in vitro, and extracts of this plant have been shown to have vasodilator properties in human experiments. In the prescription containing Ephedra sinica, which is used for asthma and coughs, the known bronchodilator effects of ephedrine from this plant fully justify this mixture as being used for asthma and coughs.

Activity Rating = +5,0,+5

GRAMINEAE

Imperata cylindrica Dried roots Activity Rating = +3,+3,0	a. For hemoptysis, epistaxis and hematuria, combine with Rehmannia glutinosa, Gardenia jasminoides and Agrimonia viscidula and decoct, or combine with Cephalanopsis segetum and Nelumbo nucifera and pound out the juice. b. For acute nephritis, decoct and use alone. c. For cough with expectoration, decoct and use alone.	Imperata cylindrica is also used in Japan as an herbal remedy for its diuretic and antiinflammatory properties (acute nephritis?). It has folkloric medicinal uses in other countries as a hemostatic, antipyretic and for arthirits. Extracts of I.cylindrica have been pharmacologically evaluated and show antiviral activity, but the following pharmacological parameters were all negative: effects on the CNS, analgesic, anticonvulsant, cardiovascular, smooth muscle effects, diuretic, anticancer, antibacterial, antiprotozoan, antifungal and hypoglycemic effects. Other workers have reported anticancer activity for this plant in animals.
Lophatherum gracile Dried whole plant Activity Rating = +4,+5	a. For fever and anxiety, decoct with Rehmannia glutinosa and Ophiopogon japonicus. b. For oligouria and bloody urine, decoct with Hocquartia manshuriensis, Glycyrrhiza uralensis and Rehmannia glutinosa.	Extracts of Lophatherum elatum, closely related to L.gracile, have been shown to elicit an antipyretic effect in rats, thus it is reasonable to assume that L.gracile would produce a similar effect.
Phragmites communis Dried rhizome or fresh root Activity Rating = 0,+4,+5	a. For fever and cough with yellow sputum, decoct alone or with Prunus armeniaca and Eriobotrya japonica. b. For lung pain and cough, decoct with Oryza sativa, watermelon seeds and Prunus persica. c. For stomach fever, vomiting and hiccups, decoct the fresh root with Nelumbo nucifera rhizomes, Pyrus malus (pear) and chestnut (Aesculus sp.).	Phragmites communis has been used as as herbal remedy for cancer.

GUTTIFERAE

√ **Hypericum japonicum*

Whole plant

a. For contusions from falls, decoct with water and wine (1:1) and take orally. Use the residue externally. Can also be combined with *Centipeda minima*, ground to a powder, and taken orally with wine.

b. For snake bite, decoct and take alone orally, or combine with *Lobelia chinensis* and *Houttuynia cordata* and decoct.

c. For febrile jaundice, decoct and take orally or combine with *Gardenia jasminoides*, *Plantago asiatica*, *Imperata cylindrica* and decoct.

d. For hernia and common cold, decoct and take orally.

Hypericum japonicum has been shown to have antitumor activity in animals. Other *Hypericum* species with antitumor activity are *H.perforatum*. *H.chinense*, *H.revolutum* and *H.erectum*. At least 17 species of *Hypericum* have shown *in vitro* antibacterial activity, and the antibacterial constituent has been identified in *Hypericum uliginosum* as uliginosin A and B (terpene quinones). Other *Hypericum* species have shown *in vitro* antifungal activity, and seven species are reported to elicit antiviral effects in vitro. Extracts of *Hypericum perforatum* show antidiarrheal, sedative, antitumor, and diuretic (active principle is the flavonoid hyperoside) activity. A new catechol derivative and hyperoside (from *H.perforatum*) have been shown to reduce capillary fragility.

Activity Rating = +5,0,+5,0

LABIATAE

Agastache rugosa Stem and leaves	a. For fever due to high temperature and humidity in summer and fall, headache, nausea, vomiting and chest congestion and diarrhea, decoct with Atractylodes lancea, Magnolia officinalis, Pinellia ternata and Perilla frutescens. b. For "weak spleen", vomiting, diarrhea, and thirst when one does not want to drink water, decoct with Pueraria pseudo-hirsuta, Codonopsis pilosula, Atractylodes macrocephala, and Saussurea lappa. c. For vomiting in pregnancy, decoct with Glycyrrhiza uralensis and Cyperus rotundus.	Agastache rugosa has been used as an herbal remedy for treating cancer outside of China and extracts of this plant have shown experimental antitumor activity in laboratory animals. It has also been used as a herbal remedy as an antiemetic. See Pinellia ternata (analgesic) See Cyperus rotundus (antiemetic)
Activity Rating = +5,+3,+5		
Ajuga decumbens Whole plant	a. For colds, fever and hypertension, decoct alone and take orally. b. For sore throat, inflammation and tonsillitis, decoct alone and take orally or triturate the fresh plant, filter and gargle then drink the filtrate. c. For bronchitis and pneumonia, decoct alone and take orally or decoct with Houttuynia cordata. d. For abscesses and snakebite, decoct alone and take orally or triturate the fresh plant with salt and apply externally. e. For inflammations and wound burns, apply externally.	Ajuga bracteosa has been used as an herbal remedy outside of China as an antipyretic, for wound healing, and as an antiinfective agent. The ecdysones, cyasterone, ecdysterone, ajugalactone, ajugasterone and ajugasterone C have been isolated from A. decumbens. The strong possibility exists that these compounds should have anti-inflammatory activity due to their unusual steroidal nature. Ajuga decumbens has been used outside of China as an anticancer remedy and A. bracteosa extracts have shown anticancer activity in animals, as well as smooth muscle relaxant properties. Ecdysones have analgesic activity in humans.
Activity Rating = 0,+4,+5,+2,+2		

*Leonurus heterophyllus Whole plant and fruit	a. For post-partum hemorrhage and menorrhagia, alone or with Prunus armeniaca fruits and black sugar. b. For menoxenia, with Angelica sinensis, Paeonia lactiflora and Saussurea lappa. c. For "liver fever," ophthalmia and "cloudy eye," the seeds of L. heterophyllus are decocted with Chrysanthemum morifolium, Cassia tora, Celosia argentea and Rehmannia glutinosa. d. For hypertension, this plant is used with other drugs.	An unidentified Leonurus species has been shown to have hemostatic activity. Although nothing pertaining to L. heterophyllus has been reported in the literature, it is apparent from the following that this species would be expected to have sedative, hypotensive, and cardiotonic activities. For example, L.sibiricus, L.glaucescens and L.deminutus have all shown sedative and hypotensive activity in animals, as well as hypotensive effects in humans. Leonurus lanatus has been shown to produce sedative effects in humans, in addition to cardiotonic effects. Leonurus cardiaca has been used as a folkloric sedative, and sedative activity as well as a hypotensive effect in normo-and hypertensive animals have been confirmed. It has been used clinically for hypertension in the USSR with good results. Similar effects are reported for L. sibiricus in the USSR. L.sibiricus also causes vasoconstriction. Leonurus tataricus also has been shown to be hypotensive in animals. Leonurus quinquelobatus has cardiotonic activity, which is attributed to the alkaloid stachydrine, and is also hemostatic. See Cassia tora (antibacterial).
Activity Rating = +4,+4,+5,+4		
Lycopus lucidus Dried whole herb	a. For amenorrhea and extravasation of blood, combine with Carthamus tinctorius, Leonurus heterophyllus, and Angelica sinensis and then decoct, or combine with Angelica sinensis,	Lycopus lucidus has been used as an herbal remedy for cancer. The related Lycopus virginicus and Lycopus europaeus have shown an antithyroid effect in animals, and

	Paeonia lactiflora and *Rehmannia glutinosa* and then decoct. b. For edema and polyuria after parturition, combine with *Stephania tetrandra* and then powder and take orally. c. For "swelling," grind the stems and leaves and use externally.	the active principle is stated to be lithospermic acid. *Lycopus virginicus* reduces blood pressure in experimental animals and has a strengthening action on the heart. *Lycopus virginicus* has sedative and cardiotonic activity.
Activity Rating = 0,0,0,+4		
Mentha arvensis Whole plant	a. For sore throat, decoct with *Glycyrrhiza uralensis*, *Platycodon grandiflorum*, *Schizonepeta tenuifolia* and *Bombyx mori*. b. For early symptoms of measles, decoct with *Forsythia suspensa*, *Arctium lappa*, *Cryptotympana atrata* and *Schizonepeta tenuifolia*. c. For the common cold, headaches, ophthalmia, cold sores, toothache and dermatitis.	*Mentha arvensis* has been used as an herbal analgesic, for cancer, and for cardiovascular disorders. The volatile oil from this plant has shown antispasmodic activity, as well as *in vitro* antibacterial and antifungal activity.
Activity Rating = +5,0,+3		
Perilla frutescens var. *crispa* Dried branches, leaves and seeds	a. For influenza or colds, decoct with *Zingiber officinale*, or decoct with *Prunus armeniaca* and *Citrus* spp. If there is chest pain, add *Cyperus rotundus*. b. For "crab" intoxication (vomiting), for colds or nausea, decoct alone and take orally. c. For nausea of pregnancy, use the branches and decoct with *Citrus* spp. and *Pinellia ternata*. d. For bronchitis, asthma, or as an expectorant, decoct with *Raphanus sativus* and *Lepidium apetalum*.	An unidentified *Perilla* species has been reported to be an effective anticancer drug in Japan. See *Pinellia ternata* (antiemetic).
Activity Rating = 0,0,+5,+4		

*Prunella vulgaris Dried fruit	a. For "liver-fire", headache, ophthalmia, vertigo, tinnitus aurium, bitter taste in the mouth, and anxiety, decoct alone and take orally or decoct with Uncaria rhynchophylla, Chrysanthemum morifolium, Cassia tora and Lamprotula leai. b. For scrofula, decoct alone and take orally or decoct with Scrophularia ningpoensis and Ostrea sp. c. For hypertension, decoct and take orally.	Nothing of chemical or pharmacological interest was found relative to Prunella species.
Activity Rating = 0,0,0		
Salvia miltiorhiza Dried root	a. For dysmenorrhea, menoxenia and blood clots remaining after labor, use alone or decoct with Angelica sinensis, Cyperus rotundus, Carthamus tinctorius and Ligusticum wallichii. b. For furunculosis and inflammation, decoct with Forsythia suspensa, Lonicera japonica, Paeonia lactiflora and Trichosanthes kirilowii. c. for palpitation and insomnia, decoct with Polygala tenuifolia, Thuja orientalis, Polygonum multiflorum and Zizyphus jujuba.	A number of novel diterpenoid quinones have been isolated from Salvia miltiorhiza, but no pharmacological effects have been attributed to them. Their chemical structure is such that it would be predicted that they would have some pharmacological activities. This species has been clinically evaluated in China for the treatment of tuberculous cystospasm, and it has a reputation in China as a useful anticancer remedy, but such effects have not been confirmed in animals. Other Salvia species have been reported to elicit a variety of biological effects in animals, including the following: anticonvulsant, sedative (volatile oil), hypotensive (volatile oil), hypoglycemic (in humans), anticancer, antiprotozoan, antiviral, diuretic (due to ursolic acid), anit-inflammatory, antipyretic, estrogenic, and antibacterial (in vitro).

* This plant was repeatedly, and presumably erroneously, referred to as Brunella vulgaris in China.

Other Salvia species are used outside of China as herbal remedies as follows: antidiarrheal, for rheumatism and, female disorders, antibiotic, CNS stimulant, choleretic, diuretic, and for wound healing. In prescription (b) paeoniflorin, which would be expected to be in Paeonia lactiflora, has been shown to exhibit anti-inflammatory activity in animals

Activity Rating = +5,+5,+5

Schizonepeta tenuifolia Dried stems and umbell flowers	a. For the common cold, initial symptoms of measles and furunculosis, decoct with Ledebouriella seseloides, Mentha arvensis and Glycyrrhiza uralensis. b. For epistaxis and bleeding after labor, grind to a powder and take orally or mix with "baby stool", or alone and take with water orally. c. For tonsillitis, decoct with Glycyrrhiza uralensis and Platycodon grandiflorum. d. For blood in feces, decoct with the flowers of Sophora japonica, Thuja orientalis and Citrus aurantium.	No information of interest was found in the literature relative to the chemical constituents and pharmacological activities of Schizonepeta tenuifolia, but extracts of Schizonepeta multifida show in vitro antibacterial activity. See Glycyrrhiza uralensis (anti-inflammatory) and Platycodon tenuifolia (antipyretic, anti-inflammatory).

Activity Raing = +5,0,+5,0

Scutellaria baicalensis Dried root	a. For high fever and dry coughs, decoct with Coptis chinensis, Glycyrrhiza uralensis, Paeonia lactiflora and Pueraria pseudo-hirsuta. b. For vomiting of blood and constipation, decoct with Gardenia jasminoides, Rheum tanguticum, Coptis chinensis and Glycyrrhiza uralensis.	Scutellaria baicalensis has been used as an herbal remedy for cancer, and this activity has been confirmed in animal studies. Extracts of this plant have been shown to be diuretic, and to elicit choleretic activity in animals. Three flavonoids isolated from this plant, i.e. baicalin, wogonin and bicalein, are the active diuretic

c. For stabilizing the fetus, decoct with _Atractylodes macrocephala_.
d. For preventing spontaneous abortion, decoct with _Atractylodes macrocephala_ and the root of _Boehmeria nivea_, as well as _Angelica sinensis_.
e. For eczema, triturate with _Phellodendron amurense_ and concentrated tea (_Camellia sinensis_), and use externally.

principles. Wogonin has also been shown to elicit _in vitro_ antibacterial effects, as have extracts of _Scutellaria baicalensis_. Extracts also show sedative and cardiotonic activity. Flavonoids from _Scutellaria baicalensis_ have shown antihistaminic activity.

See _Rheum tanguticum_ [prescription (b)] (cathartic).

Activity Rating = +4,+5,+4,0,0

LAURACEAE

Cinnamomum cassia Dried bark and twigs	a. For dysuria, lumbago in old men, combine with *Aconitum carmichaeli*, *Dioscorea batatas*, *Rehmannia glutinosa* and *Cornus officinalis* and decoct. b. For stomach ache, take the powder orally. c. For dyspepsia and as an aperient, the bark with *Codonopsis pilosula*, *Atractylodes macrocephala* and *Zingiber officinale* and then decoct. d. For amenorrhea and dysmenorrhea, combine with *Cyperus rotundus*, *Artemisia argyi* and *Angelica sinensis* and decoct. e. For the common cold, headache and fever, combine the twigs with *Paeonia lactiflora*, *Glycyrrhiza uralensis*, *Zingiber officinale* and *Zizyphus jujuba* and decoct.	*Cinnamomum cassia* has been reported as an herbal remedy for cancer as well as for hypertension, stomach ailments, and as a photosensitizer. Experimentally, *Cinnamomum cassia* extracts have shown *in vitro* antifungal activity as well as antibacterial activity. The volatile oil from this plant has shown antiviral activity, as well as hypotensive and cardiovascular effects. Cinnamaldehyde, which is known to be present in *Cinnamomum cassia*, has been shown to have sedative activity in mice, is hypothermic, and antipyretic. See *Dioscorea batatas* (anti-inflammatory).
Activity Rating = +5,+3,0,+5,+5		
Lindera strychnifolia Dried root	a. For tympanites of the abdomen and chest, decoct with *Cyperus rotundus*, and *Saussurea lappa*. b. For scrotal hernia, decoct with *Foeniculum vulgare* and *Citrus* sp. c. For dysmenorrhea, decoct with *Angelica sinensis*, *Corydalis bulbosa* and *Paeonia lactiflora*.	No pharmacologic data were found for *Lindera* species that correlate with the stated uses of *L. strychnifolia* in Chinese medicine. In prescription (c) *Paeonia lactiflora* would be expected to relax uterine muscle since *P. albiflora* has shown this effect in animals.
Activity Rating = 0,0,+5		

LEGUMINOSAE

Amblytropis multiflora Dried whole plant	a. For "sloughing ulcers" and dermatitis, decoct with Forsythia suspensa and Chrysanthemum morifolium and take orally. Also, the fresh plant can be triturated with the leaves of Hibiscus mutabilis, together with a little salt, and applied externally. b. For snake bite, triturate the fresh plant and take the filtrate orally. c. For jaundice and epistaxis, decoct the fresh plant and take orally with honey. d. For appendicitis, decoct with Taraxacum mongolicum, Portulaca oleracea, Scutellaria baicalensis and Salvia miltiorhiza.	Nothing relative to the chemical constituents or pharmacological effects of Amblytropis multiflora was found in the literature. See Forsythia suspensa (anticancer).

Activity Rating = +5,+3,0,0,+5

Astragalus membranaceus Dried root	a. For anorexia, weakness, rectocele and prolapse of the uterus, combine with Codonopsis pilosula, Atractylodes foetida, and then decoct. b. For the common cold, combine with Ledebouriella seseloides, and Atractylodes macrocephala and decoct. c. For edema and oligouria, combine with Stephania tetrandra, Atractylodes macrocephala and Glycyrrhiza uralensis and then decoct. d. For arthritic pain and numbness, combine with Cinnamomum cassia, Zingiber officinale, Paeonia lactiflora, Zizyphus jujuba and decoct, or combine with Angelica sinensis and decoct.	Extracts of Astragalus membranaceus have shown in vitro antibacterial effects, as well as hypoglycemic activity in animals. As an herbal remedy, this plant has been used for high blood pressure and for nephritis.

Activity Rating = +4,0,+2,+4

Cassia tora	a. For "liver fire", earache and vertigo, decoct with Uncaria rhynchophylla, Prunella vulgaris, Gentiana scabra and Lamprotula leai. b. For ophthalmia and photophobia, decoct with Equisetum hiemale, Tribulus terrestris and Chrysanthemum morifolium. c. For constipation, decoct with Cannabis sativa and Trichosanthes kirilowii.	Cassia tora has been used as an herbal remedy outside of China as an antifungal agent, for high blood pressure, as an insecticide, laxative, antipyretic, antibacterial, anthelmintic, anticonvulsant, and for cancer. Experimentally, extracts of Cassia tora have shown in vitro antibacterial and antiviral effects, and in animals, smooth muscle relaxant effects. Cathartic activity of Cassia tora is due to the presence of anthraquinones, which have been isolated and identified. An oxytocic principle has been isolated from this species, but has not been identified. The antibacterial effect of this plant can be attributed to the anthraquinones. See Gentiana macrophylla (choleretic). In prescription (c) Trichosanthes kirilowii would be predicted to contain cucurbitacins, which are known to have a cathartic effect.
Activity Rating = +5,+5,+4		
*Glycyrrhiza uralensis Dried roots	a. For weakness and anorexia, decoct with Codonopsis pilosula, Atractylodes macrocephala, Poria cocos. b. For cough with expectoration, dizziness and palpitation, decoct with Citrus sp., Pinellia ternata and Poria cocos. c. For laryngopharyngitis and cough, decoct with Platycodon grandiflorum, Mentha arvensis and Arctium lappa.	The following compounds have been isolated from Glycyrrhiza species that have been shown to have anti-inflammatory properties in experimental animals: quercetin, rutin liquiritin, liquiritigenin, licurazid, liquiritone, isoliquiritigenin, isoliquiritin, neoliquiritin and neoisoliquiritin (all flavonoids), as well as the triterpenoid glycyrrhetic acid.

	d. For bleeding hemorrhoids, decoct with Lonicera japonica, Chrysanthemum indicum and Taraxacum mongolicum.	The latter compound has also shown antibacterial activity in vitro, as well as antitussive activity. In 1973 a publication from the PRC reported on the clinical evaluation of G.uralensis in burn patients. Aside from a number of marked pharmacological effects, including corticosteroid-like activities, for the constituents of Glycyrrhiza species, glycyrrhizin (a triterpenoid glycoside) is responsible for the licorice-like taste of these species, and it is also 50 times sweeter than sugar. Undoubtedly these latter properties account for the widespread use of G.uralensis in many polyprescriptions. In prescription (c), platycodin from Platycodon grandiflorum has been shown to have expectorant properties in animal tests. See Codonopsis pilosula (stimulation of rbc formation, etc.).

Activity Rating = +5,0,+5,+2

Psoralea corylifolia Dried ripe fruit	a. For "spleen weakness," impotency, and premature ejaculations, grind with Cuscuta chinensis and Juglans nigra and take with wine or a salt solution. b. For polyuria or enuresis, grind the ripe fruit and take with water. c. For "spleen weakness" and lumbago, decoct or fry with Cinnamomum cassia and Achyranthes bidentata. d. For "spleen weakness" and diarrhea, decoct with Schisandra chinensis.	Extracts of Psoralea corylifolia have been shown to produce photosensitization in humans.

Evodia rutaecarpa, Zingiber officinale and Zizyphus jujuba.

Activity Rating = 0,0,+4,0

Pueraria pseudo-hirsuta

(syn. Pueraria lobata)
Dried tuberous root and flowers

a. For early symptoms of measles, decoct with Cimicifuga foetida Glycyrrhiza uralensis and Arctium lappa.
b. For the common cold and for thirst, decoct with Scutellaria baicalensis and Glycyrrhiza uralensis.
c. For the initial stages of fever and for sweating, decoct with Cinnamomum cassia, Glycyrrhiza uralensis and Paeonia lactiflora.
d. For thirst due to alcoholism, decoct alone.

Extracts of an unspecified Pueraria species have shown antispasmodic activity, and the active principle has been identified as the isoflavone daidzein. Pueraria thunbergiana extracts have shown anti-inflammatory activity in vitro. Pueraria mirifica has yielded the estrogenic substance mirificin. Pueraria hirsuta (presumably closely related to P.pseudo-hirsuta), has been found to contain choline, allantoin and an unidentified cholinergic substance. Other components of this plant have shown parasympathomimetic activity, as well as choleretic activity, and they lower blood pressure. Extracts also inhibit choline esterase. During our trip to the PRC we were told that P.pseudo-hirsuta decoctions were used to treat patients for neck stiffness, and for hypertension.
In prescription (c), paeoniflorin from Paeonia albiflora, has been shown to have marked hypothermic activity in animals.

Activity Rating = 0,0,+4,0

Sophora flavescens

Dried root

a. For diarrhea and hemorrhoidal hemorrhaging, decoct and use alone, or decoct with Saussurea lappa and Glycyrrhiza uralensis.

Sophora flavescens has been used as an herbal remedy for cancer and has shown in vitro antibacterial effects. The plant is also used as an herbal.

	b. For jaundice, decoct with *Gentiana scabra* and *Gardenia jasminoides*. c. For *Trichomonas vaginalis* infections, decoct alone and use as a douche.	remedy for diarrhea. See also *Sophora japonica* and *Sophora subprostrata*. See also *Gardenia jasminoides* (choleretic).
Activity Rating = +5,+4,0		
Sophora japonica Dried flower bud, flowers and fruits	a. For hemorrhoids, decoct with *Thuja orientalis*, *Schizonepeta tenuifolia* and *Citrus aurantium*, or grind with *Sanguisorba officinalis*, *Angelica sinensis*, *Scutellaria baicalensis* and *Ledebouriella seseloides*. b. For hypertension, use with other antihypertensives. c. For hemorrhoidal pain, grind with *Sophora flavescens*, then triturate with water and use externally.	*Sophora japonica* has been used outside of China as a herbal remedy for hypertension, and it contains several known antitumor pyrrolizidine alkaloids. See also *Sophora subprostrata* and *Sophora flavescens*.
Activity Rating = +5,+4,+3,0		
Sophora subprostrata Dried root	a. For laryngitis, decoct and take alone or decoct with *Arctium lappa*, *Scrophularia ningpoensis*, *Platycodon grandiflorum* and *Glycyrrhiza uralensis*. b. For coughs and sore throat, decoct with *Peucedanum praeruptorum*, *Eriobotrya japonica*, *Platycodon grandiflorum* and *Glycyrrhiza uralensis*. c. Can be used for gum inflammation, acute bile duct inflammation, and jaundice. Use externally for dermatitis and inflammation.	*Sophora subprostrata* has yielded the antitumor alkaloids matrine and oxymatrine, as well as the antitumor agent sophajaponicin. Sophoradochromene, also from this plant, has been shown to have antiulcer properties in rats. See also *Sophora japonica* and *Sophora flavescens*. See *Platycodon grandiflorum* (laryngitis).
Activity Rating = +5,+5,0		

√*Spatholobus suberectus* Dried stem	a. For amenorrhea and abdominal pain, decoct with *Rehmannia glutinosa*, *Angelica sinensis*, *Paeonia lactiflora* and *Ligusticum wallichii*. b. For waist and knee pain, decoct with *Acanthopanax gracilistylis* (or *Periploca sepium*), *Angelica sinensis*, *Rehmannia glutinosa* and *Notopterygium incisum*. c. For leukopenia, use in conjunction with other tonics.	Nothing of value concerning the chemical constituents or pharmacological effects could be found relative to *Spatholobus suberectus*.

Activity Rating = 0,0,0

LILIACEAE

Anemarrhena asphodeloides Dried rhizome	a. For congestive fever, thirst and excess sweating, combine with calcium sulfate, Oryza sativa, Glycyrrhiza uralensis and decoct. b. For "eruptions," combine with calcium sulfate, Oryza sativa, Glycyrrhiza uralensis, Scrophularia ningpoensis and Rehmannia glutinosa and decoct. c. For dry throat and hacking cough, combine with Artemisia apiaca, Stemona sessilifolia and decoct. d. For premature ejaculations, vertigo, tinnitis aurium and lumbago, combine with Rehmannia glutinosa, Chinemys reevesii and decoct or grind to a powder and take orally, or combine with Rehmannia glutinosa, Cornus officinalis and Dioscorea batatas and decoct or grind to a powder and take orally.	Anemarrhena asphodeloides has been used as an herbal remedy for treating hypertension and diabetes. Extracts have shown hypoglycemic activity in animals, as well as anticancer effects. Extracts of this plant would be expected to elicit anti-inflammatory effects due to the presence of steroidal saponins, which are known to show this type of activity in animals; thus the use of this plant in Traditional Chinese medicine for treating lumbago may be justified. See Dioscorea batatas (anti-inflammatory).

Activity Rating = +5,0,0,0,0,+5

Asparagus cochinchinensis Dried tuberous root	a. For hacking cough and thirst, combine with Ophiopogon japonicus, Glehnia littoralis and decoct, or combine with Ophiopogon japonicus and decoct. Add honey and take orally. b. For spitting of blood, combine with Paeonia lactiflora, Rehmannia glutinosa and Nelumbo nucifera and decoct. c. For constipation after fever and for thirst, combine with Rehmannia glutinosa, Scrophularia ningpoensis,	The only report on the pharmacological activity of Asparagus cochinchinensis is that it has antitumor activity in animals. Other Asparagus species have been reported to elicit the following pharmacological activities in animals: diuretic, anticancer, anthelmintic, antipyretic, smooth muscle relaxant, antioxytocic, galactagogue, and in vitro antibacterial activity. Folkloric uses outside of China for Asparagus species include: analgesic, choleretic, antipyretic,

	Cannabis sativa and Angelica sinensis and decoct.	antibacterial, anthelmintic, sedative, cardiotonic, antidiarrheal, diuretic, aphrodisiac, anti-inflammatory, contraceptive and hypoglycemic.
Activity Rating = 0,0,0,0		
Fritillaria cirrhosa Dried bulb	a. For chronic cough, hacking, chronic bronchitis and tuberculosis, grind alone with Anemarrhena asphodeloides (or Bletilla striata) and take orally, or decoct with Glehnia littoralis, and Ledebouriella seseloides.	Although no reports could be found on the biological activities of F. cirrhosa, alkaloids and extracts of other Fritillaria species, which would most likely also be found in F.cirrhosa, have interesting pharmacological effects. For example, imperialine, a steroid alkaloid of F. imperialis, relaxes smooth muscle in a manner similar to papaverine. A similar alkaloid, fritimine, also relaxes smooth muscle. Verticine, verticilline, fritillarine and fritilline, all from F.verticillata, have local anesthetic activity. Alginine, an alkaloid from F.sewerzowii, has effects similar to cocaine, whereas peimunine, from an unidentified Chinese Fritillaria species, has effects similar to atropine. Tuliposide A, a lactonic glycoside from F.imperialis and several other Fritillaria species, has shown antiallergic properties in animals, which could act to dry nasal secretions and explain the use of F.cirrhosa in treating "hacking coughs". Alkaloid extracts from F. imperialis have shown respiratory stimulant activity in animals.
Activity Rating = +4,+4		

Fritillaria thunbergii (syn. Fritillaria verticillata) Dried bulb	a. For the common cold and coughs with expectoration, combine with Prunus armeniaca, Cynanchum stauntoni and Aster tataricus and decoct. b. For swellings, combine with Scrophularia ningpoensis, Prunella vulgaris and Ostrea spp. and decoct or grind to a powder and take orally. c. For mastitis, combine with Taraxacum mongolicum, Lonicera japonica and Forsythia suspensa and decoct. d. For stomach ache and hyperacidity, combine with Sepia esculenta and then decoct, or powder and take orally.	Fritillaria thunbergii has been used as an herbal remedy for cancer. Peimine and peimisidine, two steroidal alkaloids have been isolated from this plant. Both of these alkaloids lower blood pressure in animals. Other steroidal alkaloids isolated from this plant include verticine (peimine), verticilline, fritillarine (verticinone) and fritilline (peimine), which all have been shown to paralyze sensory nerves and respiration, cause vasoconstriction and cardiac and motor paralysis in frogs. Fritimine (peimine) lowers blood pressure in anesthetized cats, temporarily depresses respiration, increases blood sugar levels in rabbits, contracts the isolated guinea pig uterus and inhibits the isolated rabbit intestine. Another alkaloid, peimunine, relaxes smooth muscle. Verticine, verticilline and fritillarine, all act on skeletal muscle, are hypertensive and relax smooth muscle. See also Fritillaria cirrhosa (smooth muscle relaxant).
Activity Rating = +4,0,0,+5		
Lilium brownii var. colchesteri Dried bulb	a. For "weakness," "fire in the body," cough, decoct with Ophiopogon japonicus, Paeonia lactiflora, Scrophularia ningpoensis and Rehmannia glutinosa. b. For "weak lungs," spitting and hemoptysis, grind with Tussilago farfara	No pharmacologic studies have been published concerning Lilium brownii, however, several species of Lilium have been shown to elicit antihistaminic as well as antibacterial effects. In prescription (a), paeoniflorin

	and eat after mixing with honey. c. For the late stages of fever, decoct alone or with Rehmannia glutinosa and Anemarrhena asphodeloides.	from Paeonia albiflora, has been shown to have marked hypothermic activity in animals. See Paeonia suffruticosa (smooth muscle relaxant).
Activity Rating = +4,0,0,		
Ophiopogon japonicus Dried tuberous root	a. For "lung and stomach weakness," sore throat and cough, decoct with Glehnia littoralis, Pinellia ternata and Glycyrrhiza uralensis. b. For cough and sore throat, decoct with Morus alba, Prunus armeniaca, Scropularia ningpoensis and Eriobotrya japonica. c. For fever (late stages), and constipation, decoct with Scrophularia ningpoensis and Rehmannia glutinosa.	The only report on the biological effects of Ophiopogon species found in the literature was that extracts of this plant (O. japonicus) show antitumor activity in animals. See Pinellia ternata (analgesic). See Prunus armeniaca (demulcent).
Activity Rating = +5,+5,0		
Paris polyphylla Dried rhizome	a. For snake bite poisoning, grind alone and take orally or decoct with Lobelia chinensis and Prunella vulgaris, and take orally. In case of constipation, add Rheum tanguticum. b. For "sloughing ulcers," triturate with vinegar and apply to affected areas. c. For scrofula, decoct with Prunella vulgaris and Semiaquilegia adoxoides.	Extracts of the related Paris formosana have been reported to be cytotoxic in vitro and to have antitumor activity in vivo (for sloughing ulcers?). Diosgenin glycosides isolated from Paris polyphylla would be expected to have anti-inflammatory activity. Rheum tanguticum contains cathartic glycosides.
Activity Rating = 0,0,+5,+4,0		

Polygonatum officinale (syn. Polygonatum glaberrium) Dried rhizome	a. For lung fever, hacking cough and dry mouth, decoct with Ophiopogon japonicus, Glehnia littoralis, Morus alba and Trichosanthes kirilowii. b. For the common cold, fever, cough and sore throat, decoct with Allium cepa, Mentha arvensis, Platycodon grandiflorum and Cynanchum atratum. c. For weakness after illness, decoct alone or with Codonopsis pilosula and Atractylodes macrocephala.	Polygonatum officinale extracts have been shown to decrease blood sugar levels in rabbits, as well as to elicit a cardiotonic effect, and to lower blood pressure. The wound-healing and anti-inflammatory active compound allantoin has been isolated from this plant. See Platycodon grandiflorum (antitussive). See Codonopsis pilosula (hematopoetic).

Activity Rating = +3,+5,+5

LORANTHACEAE

Viscum coloratum

Dried stems and leaves

a. For rheumatic pain, sore knee and waist, decoct with Angelica pubescens and A.sinensis.
b. For "fetus-leaking," "fetus-moving" and spontaneous abortion, decoct with Dipsacus asper, Angelica sinensis and Paeonia lactiflora.
c. For hypertension, decoct alone or with Clerodendrum trichotomum and Uncaria rhynchophylla.

No work has been found concerning Viscum coloratum. However, it is well known that most Viscum species contain toxic proteins. Viscum album has shown anticancer and cytotoxic effects in animals and in humans, and the active principles are a group of proteins known as viscotoxins. In addition, V. album extracts have shown histaminic activity, and histamine, choline and acetycholine have been isolated from this plant. Further, gamma amino-butyric acid has been shown to be a hypotensive ingredient in V. album. Extracts of V. album have shown hypotensive activity in animals, and such extracts have been shown to slow the pulse and depress the heart. Extracts also stimulate the isolated intestine and uterus, and have cholinomimetic activity. Several triterpenes have been isolated from V.album that have been shown to have anti-inflammatory activity in laboratory animals.

See Uncaria rhynchophylla (hypotensive).

Activity Rating = +5,0,+5

MAGNOLIACEAE

*Magnolia officinalis Dried stem bark, root bark and flower	a. For dyspepsia, anorexia, nausea, vomiting and diarrhea, decoct with Atractylodes lancea, Citrus spp. and Glycyrrhiza uralensis. b. For flatulence and constipation, decoct with Citrus aurantium and Rheum tanguticum. c. For coughs and abdominal tympanites, decoct with Prunus armeniaca, Paeonia lactiflora and Cinnamomum cassia.	Nothing could be found in the literature concerning the chemical constituents or pharmacological activities of Magnolia species. Rheum tanguticum would be the active cathartic principle in prescription (b) due to its known anthraquinones. In prescription (c), Prunus armeniaca would contribute to the use of this mixture for coughs due to the presence of pectin, and Paeonia species are known to have antispasmodic and antibacterial activity.

Activity Rating = 0,+5,+5

MALVACEAE

Abutilon avicennae Dried ripe seed Activity Rating = +3,+3,+4	a. For dysuria, decoct with talc, and Agastache rugosa. b. For dysentery, grind the powder and take orally. c. Grind with honey and use externally for keratitis.	Abutilon avicennae contains alkaloids and has been used as an herbal remedy outside of China for dysentery, as a diuretic and as an antipyretic. Other species having herbal remedial uses outside of China include the following: A.laxiflorum as an analgesic, A. mauritianum for asthma and as an antipyretic in malaria, as well as for fungal diseases and for allergies, A.americanum for cancer, A.indicum for asthma, dysentery, for bladder or kidney disorders, as an aphrodisiac, and as an antibacterial, A.theophrasti for use in dysentery, as a diuretic and for fevers, and A.molle for stomach ailments. Experimentally A.theophrasti has shown CNS depressant activity in mice, A.indicum has shown anticonvulsant, smooth muscle relaxant, antitussive antidiarrheal, uterine stimulant and antibacterial activity, as well as antipyretic activity. Abutilon asiaticum has shown anticancer activity in animals.
Hibiscus mutabilis Dried leaves and flowers Activity Rating = 0,0,0,+4	a. For inflammation, pound out the juice and use externally, or combine the powdered leaves with oil or tea extract and use externally. b. For snakebite, use as above. c. For burns.	A related species, Hibiscus moschatus is used in Mexico as a remedy for snakebite. Hibiscus mutabilis has been reported as a folkloric remedy for cancer. Hibiscus species contain large amounts of mucilages, which would act as emollients for burns.
Malva verticillata (syn. Malva chinensis) Seed Activity Rating = 0,0,0	a. Same uses as described for Abutilon avicennae.	Malva verticillata has been used as an herbal remedy for cancer.

MELIACEAE

Melia toosendan Dried ripe fruit and stem bark	a. For chest and abdominal pain, decoct with Corydalis bulbosa. b. For female abdominal and chest pain and tympanites of abdomen during the cycle, decoct the fruit with Angelica sinensis, Paeonia lactiflora, Carthamus tinctorius and Bupleurum scorzoneraefolium. c. For tinea infections, grind the fruit with lard and apply externally once daily for 7-10 days. d. For abdominal pain caused by ascariasis, decoct the root bark alone and take orally with sugar.	Nothing has been found in the literature relative to M.toosendan. The majority of information on this genus of plants concerns M.azadirachta, which has yielded a number of novel limonoids, whose biological properties have not yet been described. **M. azadirachta has shown smooth muscle relaxant, anticancer and hypoglycemic effects, and the volatile oil of this plant inhibits both Gram positive and Gram negative bacteria in vitro. Melia indica has yielded the compound nimbin, which shows spermicidal activity.** See Corydalis bulbosa (analgesic).

Activity Rating = +5,+4,0,0

MENISPERMACEAE

Stephania tetrandra Dried root Activity Rating = 0,+5	a. Same uses as for Aristolochia westlandi.	Tetrahydropalmatine is present in most members of the genus Stephania, and this alkaloid is known to have sedative, tranquilizing and analgesic activity in humans.

MORACEAE

Broussonetia papyrifera Dried ripe fruit	a. For impotency, decoct alone and take orally. b. For tinea infections, use the latex from the bark and apply externally, or use in the form of a tincture externally. c. The leaves and bark can be used for vomiting of blood, diarrhea, dysentery, rheumatism and nephritis.	Broussonetia papyrifera has been used as an herbal remedy outside of China for cancer, for female disorders, and for nephritis. Extracts of this plant have shown insect moulting hormone activity.
Activity Rating = 0,0,+3		
Morus alba Dried leaves, roots, twigs and fruits.	a. For the common cold, headache, and coughs, combine with Chrysanthemum morifolium and Mentha arvensis and decoct. b. For ophthalmia, prepare a decoction from the leaves and apply externally. c. For coughs, combine with Glycyrrhiza uralensis, Lycium chinense and decoct. d. For edema and oligouria, combine with Areca catechu, Poria cocos, Citrus spp. and Zingiber officinale and decoct. e. For dizziness and insomnia, combine with the fruit of Ligustrum lucidum and Eclipta prostrata and decoct. f. For constipation in old men, prepare a decoction from the fruits, or combine with Sesamum indicum and decoct. g. For arm ache, prepare a decoction from the twigs.	Morus alba has been used as an herbal remedy for cancer, coughs, diarrhea, and as an anthelmintic. Experimentally extracts of this plant have shown hormonal activity, i.e. acceleration of the growth of immature rats in feeding experiments, as well as hypoglycemic activity in animals. Antifungal activity has been shown for extracts of Morus alba by in vitro experiments. See Glycyrrhiza uralensis (antitussive).
Activity Rating = 0,0,+5,0,0,0,+3		

NYMPHAEACEAE

Nelumbo nucifera

Dried leaves, fruits, rhizome, receptacle, sprout, stamen and flowers.

a. For sunstroke or dizziness, decoct the leaves and combine with Artemisia apiacea and Glycyrrhiza uralensis, and talc decoct.
b. For diarrhea, add Atractylodes lancea, and Atractylodes macrocephala and decoct.
c. For dysentery, combine with Codonopsis pilosula, Acorus gramineus, and Coptis chinensis and decoct.
d. For congestive fever, dizziness, restlessness, thirst and odontorrhagia, combine with Scrophularia ningpoensis, Ophiopogon japonicus, and Forsythia suspensa and decoct.
e. For vomiting of blood, combine with Imperata cylindrica, and Rehmannia glutinosa and decoct.
f. For menorrhagia, combine the receptacle with Rubia cordifolia, Typha latifolia and Cephalanopsis segetum and decoct.
g. For premature ejaculations, decoct the flower or combine with Rosa laevigata and decoct.

The following alkaloids have been isolated from Nelumbo nucifera: dehydroroemerine, dehydronuciferine, dehydroanonaine, N-methylisococlaurine, roemerine, nuciferine, anonaine, pronuciferine, N-nornuciferine, nornuciferine, armepavine and N-methylcoclaurine, liriodenine, D-methylcoclaurine,-nornuciferine, isoliniensine, lotusine, neferine,.1-(p-hydroxybenzyl)-6,7-dihydroxy-1,2,3,4-tetrahydroisoquinoline, methylcorypalline, lotusine, N-norarempavine and oxoushinsunine. This plant has been used as an herbal remedy for stomach disorders and for cancer. In animals, extracts of this plant have shown antitumor properties, and the alkaloid oxoushinsunine is cytotoxic. The alkaloids nuciferine and nornuciferine have shown antispasmodic activity in animals.

See Coptis chinensis (diarrhea).

Activity Rating = 0,0,+5,0,0,0,0

OLEACEAE

Forsythia suspensa Dried fruit	a. For fever and headache, decoct with Lonicera japonica, Mentha arvensis, Schizonepeta tenuifolia, Glycyrrhiza uralensis. b. For sore throat, decoct with Scrophularia ningpoensis, Isatis tinctoria and Rehmannia glutinosa. c. For "heat spots" and "sloughing ulcers," decoct with Taraxacum mongolicum and Chrysanthemum indicum. d. For scrofula, decoct with Prunella vulgaris, Scrophularia ningpoensis and Ostrea sp.	**Forsythia suspensa has a folkloric reputation as a cancer remedy ("sloughing ulcer"?) and has been shown to have antitumor activity in laboratory animals.** Extracts of this plant have also been used outside of China as a folkloric antibiotic remedy (sore throat?). Unspecified Forsythia species have been shown to relax smooth muscle in humans, and are used in the treatment of diphtheria in China (PRC). See Isatis tinctoria (analgesic).
Activity Rating = +3,+5,+3,0		
Fraxinus rhynchophylla Dried bark	a. For diarrhea, decoct with Pulsatilla chinensis, Coptis chinensis and Phellodendron amurense. b. For ophthalmia, decoct alone and use externally as an eye wash. c. For acute hepatitis, decoct with Artemisia capillaris, Taraxacum mongolicum and Rheum tanguticum.	Only one report has been published on this species. This is a recent report on the effects of F.rhynchophyllus decoctions in acute bacillary dysentery in children, which originated from the PRC. However, several other reports have been published elsewhere on the in vitro antibacterial effects of several related Fraxinus species, and F.japonicus has been shown to have **anti-inflammatory activity (ophthalmia?)** in laboratory animals. Fraxinus ornus has a folkloric reputation outside of China as a remedy for diarrhea. See Coptis chinensis (diarrhea). See Taraxacum mongolicum (choleretic).
Activity Rating = +5,+5,+5		

Ligustrum lucidum

Dried ripe fruit

a. For "weak liver" and kidneys, tinnitus aurium and vertigo, decoct with Rehmannia glutinosa, Paeonia lactiflora, Lycium chinense and Chrysanthemum morifolium, or triturate with the above drugs and eat with the help of light salt soup.

b. For "weakness," fever, sore wrist and knee, and habitual constipation in old men, grind with Eclipta prostrata, and Morus alba and take with water, or decoct with Polygonum multiflorum, Ophiopogon japonicus, Chinemys (Geoclemys) reevesii, and Rehmannia glutinosa.

Ligustrum lucidum extracts have shown antitumor activity in animals, and a new iridoid glucoside, nuezhenide, has been isolated from this plant, but no biological activities have been attributed to it. On the other hand, related species show interesting biological activities. Ligustrum japonicum extracts show antiulcer activity in animals, decrease blood pressure, and show antibacterial activity. The latter activity is probably due to the fatty acids known to be present in many Ligustrum species. Interesting is the report of the presence of cinchonidine, cinchonine and dihydrocinchonine in L. vulgare, since if these known antipyretic alkaloids are present in L. lucidum, it could explain why this plant is useful for fevers in Chinese medicine.

See Paeonia suffruticosa (antidiuretic)
See Polygonum multiflorum (anti-inflammatory).

Activity Rating = +4,+3,+4

ORCHIDACEAE

Bletilla striata Dried tubers	a. For coughs, chest pain, and hemoptysis, decoct with *Platycodon grandiflorum* and take orally with sugar, or decoct with *Agrimonia viscidula*, *Nelumbo nucifera* and *Eriobotrya japonica*. b. For gastrorrhagia and enterorrhagia, grind to a powder and take orally or grind with *Sanguisorba officinalis* and take orally. c. For abscesses and inflammation, decoct with *Lonicera japonica*, *Forsythia suspensa*, *Trichosanthes kirilowii* and *Pinellia ternata* and take orally, or grind the fresh root with salt and apply externally. d. For wounds and external bleeding, grind to a powder with calcium sulfate and use externally. e. For chapped skin (feet and hands), grind to a powder, add water, and use externally.	Nothing was found in the literature relative to the pharmacological effects or chemical constituents of *Bletilla striata*. See *Platycodon grandiflorum* (antitussive) See *Lonicera japonica* (antibacterial).
Activity Rating = +5,0,0,0,+5,0,0		
Dendrobium hancockii Dried stem	a. For fever and thirst, combine with *Ophiopogon japonicus*, *Trichosanthes kirilowii* and *Rehmannia glutinosa* and decoct. b. For cough and thirst, combine with *Ophiopogon japonicus*, *Glehnia littoralis* and *Polygonatum officinale* and decoct.	Nothing of value was found in the literature relative to the chemical constituents or pharmacological effects of *Dendrobium hancockii*.
Activity Rating = 0,0		
Gastrodia elata Dried tuber	a. For fever, combine with *Buthus martensi*, *Morus alba*, *Chrysanthemum morifolium* and *Uncaria rhynchophylla*	Nothing of value could be found in the literature relative to the chemical constituents or pharmacological

and decoct.
b. For numbness, combine with *Angelica sinensis*, *Cyathula capitata*, *Notopterygium incisum* and *Chaenomeles lagenaria* and then decoct with wine and water.

effects of *Gastrodia* species.

Activity Rating = 0,0

PAEONIACEAE

Paeonia lactiflora Dried root	a. For menoxenia and dysmenorrhea, decoct with Angelica chinensis, Rehmannia glutinosa, Cyperus rotundus and Ligusticum wallichii. b. For "convulsions of excretion muscle" (diarrhea?), decoct with Glycyrrhiza uralensis. c. For diarrhea, decoct with Glycyrrhiza uralensis and Scutellaria baicalensis. d. For "liver-fire," headache and vertigo, decoct with Morus alba, Chrysanthemum morifolium, Uncaria rhynchophylla and Rehmannia glutinosa.	See comments under Paeonia suffruticosa. See Scutellaria baicalensis (antibacterial).
Activity Rating = +5,0,+5,0		
Paeonia suffruticosa Dried root bark	a. For fever-induced vomiting of blood, decoct with Rehmannia glutinosa, Scrophularia ningpoensis and Paeonia lactiflora. b. For fatigue-induced night fever, decoct with Lycium chinense, Artemisia apiacea and Anemarrhena asphodeloides. c. For initial period of appendicitis, decoct with Rheum tanguticum, Prunus persica and watermelon seed. d. For amenorrhea, decoct with Angelica sinensis, Cyathula capitata and Cinnamomum cassia.	Paeonia suffruticosa has been reported to have antitumor activity in animals, as have several other Paeonia species. There are several reports in the literature referring to a "Paeonia albiflora" that is frequently mentioned as being used in Chinese medicine. The possibility exists that P.suffruticosa is synonymous with P.albiflora or that P. lactiflora is synonymous with P.albiflora. In any event, they are all so similar that activities shown by one would be expected for the others. An active principle, paeoniflorin, has been isolated from P.albiflora, and it has been shown in animals to have **antispasmodic, anti-inflammatory, hypotensive (peripheral vasodilator), and smooth muscle relaxant effects of both rat stomach and uterus, antidiuretic**

effects, marked hypothermic effects, and weak anticonvulsant activity. Paeoniflorin has been shown to be synergistic in its action when combined with a *Glycyrrhiza* extract, thus substantiating the Chinese practice of often combining *Paeonia* and *Glycyrrhiza* in prescriptions. The related *P.moutan*, which is stated to be used in Chinese prescriptions for appendicitis, has been shown to inhibit Gram positive organisms *in vitro*, and the active constituent has been identified as paeonol (2'-hydroxy-4'-methoxyacetophenone). *Paeonia officinalis* extracts have been shown to exert an anticonvulsant effect in animals, and *P.moutan* extracts are sedative, anticonvulsant, and antipyretic in animals, and the active principle has been shown to be paeonol. A number of *Paeonia* species are used as folkloric sedative remedies outside of China.

Activity Rating = 0,+4,+5,0

PALMAE

√ _Areca catechu_ Dried ripe seed and pericarp	a. For ascariasis, decoct the seed and take orally. b. For diarrhea, combine with _Saussurea lappa_, _Phellodendron amurense_, _Citrus aurantium_ and _Rheum tanguticum_ and decoct. c. For dyspepsia, combine with _Crataegus pinnatifida_ or _Crataegus cuneata_ and decoct. d. For edema and oligouria, combine with _Citrus_ spp., _Poria cocos_, _Morus alba_ and _Zingiber officinale_ and decoct.	The anthelmintic activity of _Areca catechu_ is well established since this plant contains the clinically effective anthelmintic alkaloid arecoline.

Activity Rating = +5,0,0,0

PAPAVERACEAE

Corydalis bulbosa (Syn. Corydalis cava)
Dried tuber

a. For dysmenorrhea, combine with Angelica sinensis, and Cinnamomum cassia and decoct or combine with Angelica sinensis, Ligusticum wallichii, Cyperus rotundus and Cocculus laurifolius and decoct.
b. For chest pains, combine with Melia toosendan and grind to a powder and take orally, or combine with Cyperus rotundus and decoct.
c. For cholecystitis, combine with Foeniculum vulgare, Citrus spp., Cocculus laurifolius and decoct.
d. For contusions from a fall, combine with Angelica sinensis and Paeonia lactiflora and decoct.

Corydalis bulbosa (C.cava) has been used as an herbal sedative.
Several Corydalis species contain the alkaloid tetrahydropalmatine, which is an effective sedative, tranquilizer and analgesic in man. Corydalis alkaloids have also been used to prevent gastric ulcer from forming in experimental animals. Bulbocapnine has been isolated from Corydalis bulbosa and this alkaloid induces catalepsy in mice at high doses, antagonizes the effects of apomorphine and d-amphetamine in standard pharmacological tests, exhibits sedative activity as shown by decreased motor activity in mice and by potentiation of pentobarbital. Bulbocapnine, however, has a short duration of action and a low therapeutic ratio. This alkaloid has also been shown to lower blood pressure and have a cardiotonic action. Corytuberine, isolated from Corydalis bulbosa, has shown anticancer activity in animals, as well as analeptic activity. Glaucine, also isolated from this plant, lowers blood pressure and has antitussive activity. Corydine from this plant also has anticancer activity and is a CNS depressant.

See Cyperus rotundus (analgesic, relax smooth muscle).
See Paeonia suffruticosa (anti-inflammatory).

Activity Rating = 0,+5,+5,+5,0,+4

PEDALIACEAE

Sesamum indicum Dried seed	a. For impotency, weakness and dizziness, triturate with Morus alba and honey. b. For constipation, triturate with honey. c. For weakness after getting well, triturate with sugar.	Sesamum indicum has been used as an herbal laxative outside of China. See Morus alba (growth stimulation).

Activity Rating = +5,+3,0

PHYTOLACCACEAE

Phytolacca esculenta

Dried root

a. For edema, constipation and dysuria, decoct alone.
b. For roundworm infestation, grind with _Areca catechu_ and _Rheum tanguticum_ and take with water.

Phytolacca esculenta has been used as an herbal remedy for nephritis. Extracts of this plant have shown diuretic activity, and the active diuretic principle has been identified as the acidic triterpenoid jaligonic acid. A pokeweed mitogen (glycoprotein) has been isolated from this plant. Extracts of this plant have also been shown to elicit antitumor activity in animals. The use of prescription (b) for roundworm infection is justified on the basis of inclusion of _Areca catechu_ which contains the clinically effective alkaloid arecoline, which has been used for years as an anthelmintic.

Activity Rating = +5,+5

PLANTAGINACEAE

√ Plantago asiatica

Dried ripe seed and whole plant

a. For edema and dysuria, decoct alone or decoct with Poria cocos, Alisma plantago-aquatica and Atractylodes macrocephala.

b. For gonorrhea, strangury, polyuria, hematuria and urolithiasis, decoct alone or with talc, Polygonum aviculare and Glycyrrhiza uralensis.

c. For lung disease, or as an antitussive or expectorant, decoct alone, or with Cynanchum stauntoni, Morus alba and Prunus armeniaca.

d. For "sloughing ulcers", grind the whole fresh plant and apply externally.

Very little information could be found relative to the chemical constituents and pharmacological activities of Plantago asiatica, but other species offer some insight as to what might be expected for this species. For example, Plantago lanceolata has been used as an herbal remedy for cancer, and extracts of Plantago lanceolata have shown anticancer activity in animals (use of Plantago asiatica for "sloughing ulcers"?). Also, the iridoid glycoside aucubin has shown antibacterial properties, and this compound is widespread in Plantago species. Plantago major var. asiatica (Plantago asiatica?) seeds have elicited a diuretic effect, characterized by an increased output of water, urea, chloride and uric acid (in 3 patients). An alcoholic extract of Plantago ovata seeds shows cholinergic effects in animal studies. Extracts of an unidentified Plantago species produced a hypocholesterolemic effect in rabbits. The seed coat of most Plantago species is well known to contain a high content of mucilage, which would act as a demulcent or emollient if applied externally, or to be effective in soothing mucous membranes in cases of cough.

Activity Rating = +5,+4,+5,+5,+4

POLYGALACEAE

√*Polygala tenuifolia* Dried root Activity Rating = +4,+4	a. For cough and excessive production of sputum, decoct with *Aster tataricus*, *Platycodon grandiflorum*, *Glycyrrhiza uralensis* and *Prunus armeniaca*. b. For palpitation, insomnia and amnesia, decoct with *Salvia miltiorhiza*, *Ophiopogon japonicus* and *Zizyphus jujuba*.	*Polygala tenuifolia* has been used as an herbal remedy for cancer, and as an antitussive. See *Platycodon grandiflorum* (antitussive). See *Salvia miltiorhiza* (sedative).

POLYGONACEAE

Polygonum aviculare

Dried whole plant

a. For dysuria, gonorrhea and hematuria, decoct alone, or decoct with *Plantago asiatica*, *Pyrrosia lingua* and *Glycyrrhiza uralensis*.
b. For diarrhea, jaundice and roundworm infection, as well as eczema of the anus, decoct alone.

Polygonum aviculare has been used as an herbal remedy for diarrhea, as an antiinfective, for female disorders, and for cancer. Experimentally, extracts have shown *in vitro* antibacterial activity and laxative activity. The latter activity is due to anthraquinones known to be present in this plant.

See also *Polygonum cuspidatum*, *Polygonum hydropiper*, *Polygonum multiflorum* and *Polygonum orientale*.

Activity Rating = +5,0

Polygonum cuspidatum

Dried root

a. For gout after labor and for rheumatoid arthritis, macerate with wine.
b. For jaundice, decoct and take alone.
c. For gonorrhea, decoct alone or decoct with *Lobelia chinensis*.

Polygonum cuspidatum extracts have been shown to produce purgative effects in laboratory animals, due to the emodin content of this plant. Extracts of this plant have also been shown to produce gonadotrophic effects, as well as antitumor effects. The latter activity is undoubtedly due to the emodin content, which is a known antitumor agent. Most *Polygonum* species examined to date have leucoanthocyanidins, which have been shown to have anti-inflammatory activity in animals, to decrease blood coaguability, to have cardiotonic effects, hypotensive effects and vasodilating effects.

See also *Polygonum aviculare*, *Polygonum hydropiper*, *Polygonum multiflorum* and *Polygonum orientale*.

Activity Rating = +4,0,+5

Polygonum hydropiper Whole plant	a. For diarrhea and dysentery, decoct alone or decoct with Portulaca oleracea and Acalypha australis. b. For skin itching, decoct alone apply externally.	Polygonum hydropiper has been used as an herbal remedy for the following: diuretic, female disorders, wound healing, contraceptive, laxative, rheumatism, anthelmintic. Experimentally, extracts of this species have shown hormonal activity. The plant has also been used as an herbal remedy for cancer. The volatile oil from this plant has been shown to contain carvone, and this terpene has shown CNS stimulant effects in mice. Most Polygonum species have leucoanthocyanidins, which have been shown to elicit antiinflammatory effects, to decrease blood coagulability, to have cardiotonic ability, hypotensive activity, and vasodilating activity. See also Polygonum aviculare, Polygonum cuspidatum, Polygonum multiflorum and Polygonum orientale.
Activity Rating = +4,+4,+4		
Polygonum multiflorum (Syn. Polygonum chinense) Dried tuberous root.	a. For "liver and spleen weakness" and vertigo, decoct with Rehmannia glutinosa, Angelica sinensis, Lycium chinense and Cuscuta chinensis. b. For scrofula, cancer and constipation, decoct the fresh root alone. c. For insomnia, decoct with Salvia miltiorhiza and the shell of Lemprotula leai.	Polygonum multiflorum (P. chinense) has been used as an herbal sedative and for cancer outside of China. In animals, extracts of this plant show antitumor activity, as well as antiprogestational activity, sedative effects and antipyretic effects. Most Polygonum species contain leucoanthocyanidins, which have

been shown to have anti-inflammatory activity, to decrease blood coagulability, to have cardiotonic, hypotensive, and vasodilatory activity.

See also *Polygonum aviculare*, *Polygonum cuspidatum*, *Polygonum hydropiper* and *Polygonum orientale*.

Activity Rating = 0,+5,+3

Polygonum orientale
(Syn. *Polygonum pilosum*)

Ripe fruit

a. For tympanites, decoct alone.
b. For hepatitis and "sloughing ulcers", decoct alone.

Polygonum orentiale (*P. pilosum*) has been used as an herbal remedy for cancer. Experimentally, extracts of this species act as a fish poison and are devoid of antifungal activity. Most *Polygonum* species have leucoanthocyanidins, which have been shown to elicit anti-inflammatory activity, to decrease blood coagulability, to elicit cardiotonic, hypotensive, and vasodilator effects.

See also *Polygonum aviculare*, *Polygonum cuspidatum*, *Polygonum hydropiper* and *Polygonum multiflorum*.

Activity Rating = 0,+4

Rheum tanguticum

Dried rhizomes of this or other species of *Rheum*

a. For intestinal or stomach fever, and constipation, decoct with Citrus *aurantium* and *Magnolia officinalis*.

b. For acute infectious hepatitis, jaundice and constipation, decoct with *Artemisia capillaris* and *Gardenia jasminoides*.

Rheum species are well known for their use as cathartics, the activity being due to the anthraquinones that are ubiquitous in this genus. Conversely, *Rheum* preparations are also useful to treat diarrhea due to the high concentration of tannins.

	c. For diarrhea, decoct with *Areca catechu*, *Saussurea lappa* and *Coptis chinensis*. d. For amenorrhea due to blood clot, decoct with *Angelica sinensis*, *Prunus persica* and *Eupolyphaga sinensis*. e. For internal hemorrhages, grind with *Angelica sinensis* and take with wine.	Apparently, in low doses, the cathartic action predominates, whereas in high doses, diarrhea is checked because of the predominant action of the tannins. Several of the active anthraquinones have been identified in *R. tanguticum*. Biological effects reported in animals for other *Rheum* species include the following: hypocholesterolemic, diuretic, hormonal, choleretic and anticancer (several anthraquinones are known to inhibit animal tumors). *In vitro*, extracts of many *Rheum* species show antibacterial, antiviral and antifungal activities, the active principles in all of these cases are anthraquinones. *Rheum palmatum* has been used outside of China as a remedy as an ecbolic. See *Coptis chinensis* (diarrhea). See *Angelica sinensis* (hemostatic)
Activity Rating = +5,+5,+5,0,+5		
Rumex crispus (Syn. *Rumex obtusifolium*) Dried root	a. For constipation, decoct alone and take orally. b. For *tinea* infections, decoct alone and apply externally or decoct alone with vinegar and apply externally, or prepare a tincture by maceration for one week and apply externally.	*Rumex crispus* contains the known cathartic and antimicrobial anthraquinones, emodin, physcion and chrysophanol, as well as rhein.
Activity Rating = +5,0		

Rumex patientia Dried root Activity Rating = +5,0	a. Same uses as for Rumex crispus.	See also Rumex crispus.
POLYPODIACEAE Dryopteris crassirhizoma Dried rhizomes Activity Rating = +5,0,0	a. For hookworm, decoct with Melia toosendan and Perilla frutescens. b. To prevent influenza, decoct alone. c. For prolonged bleeding after labor, decoct with Paeonia suffruticosa and Nelumbo nucifera.	Filicic acid and related compounds are present in all Dryopteris species of plants investigated to date. Virtually all of the Dryopteris species are used throughout the world as anthelmintic remedies, not only by the laiety, but even by some physicians today in the United States (D. filix-mas). Filicic acid derivatives are known to be the active anthelmintic constituents.
Pteris multifida Whole plant Activity Rating = +5,0,0	a. For dysentery, decoct alone and take orally or decoct with Portulaca oleracea, Euphorbia humifusa and Polygonum aviculare. b. For jaundice, decoct alone and take orally. c. For breast pain, decoct with Taraxacum mongolicum	Nothing of value could be found in the literature regarding the chemical constituents or pharmacological activities that would support the uses for this plant in Traditional Chinese medicine. See Polygonum aviculare (antibacterial).
Pyrrosia lingua Dried whole plant Activity Rating = +5	a. For dysuria, polyuria and strangury, decoct with Plantago asiatica and talc. In case of hematuria, add Cephalanopsis segetum.	Pyrrosia lingua has shown insect moulting activity. Other Pyrrosia species have shown sedative and antispasmodic effects in animals. See Plantago asiatica (diuretic).

POLYPORACEAE

Grifola umbellata Dried sclerotium	a. For dysuria and edema, combine with Poria cocos, Alisma plantago-aquatica and talc and decoct. b. For polyuria, strangury and urethritis, combine with Hocquartia manshuriensis, Polygonum aviculare and Plantago asiatica and decoct. c. For leucorrhea, decoct and use alone as a douche.	An ethanol extract of Grifola frondosa was reported active in inhibiting the Ehrlich ascities sarcoma in mice. See Polygonum aviculare (antibacterial).
Activity Rating = +3,+5,0		
Poria cocos Dried whole fungus	a. For spleen disorders and weak stomach, use ground or decoct with Codonopsis pilosula, Atractylodes macrocephala and Glycyrrhiza uralensis, or decoct with Citrus sp., Codonopsis pilosula, Atractylodes macrocephala and Dioscorea batatas. b. For edema and dysuria, decoct with Grifola umbellata, Alisma plantago-aquatica and Atractylodes macrocephala. c. For "weak spleen," or as an antitussive and expectorant, decoct with Citrus sp., Pinellia ternata and Glycyrrhiza uralensis. d. For anxiety, amnesia, insomnia and palpitation, decoct with Polygala tenuifolia, Prunus armeniaca (kernel) and Schisandra chinensis.	The only biological effect reported in the literature for Poria cocos is that it has confirmed antitumor activity in animals and in humans. The active principle has been shown to be a polysaccharide (pachyman). Poria cocos was used previously as a folkloric remedy to treat cancer. Extracts of P. cocos have been used outside of China as folkloric choleretic and diuretic remedies. The experimental results for P. cocos do not appear to justify its various uses in Chinese medicine.
Activity Rating = 0,0,+3,+5,0		

PORTULACACEAE

√ Portulaca oleracea

Whole plant

a. For dysentery, decoct alone and take orally or pulverize and take the resulting juice with wine.
b. For "sloughing ulcers", mix with salt and use externally.
c. For eczema and dermatitis, triturate the whole fresh plant and apply externally, or decoct alone and apply externally, or decoct with Clerodendrun trichotomum and apply externally.

Portulaca oleracea has been used for a variety of illnesses as an herbal remedy, including use as a diuretic, for rheumatism and female disorders, for cancer, as a sedative, analgesic, cardiotonic, antipyretic, for urinary disorders, as an anthelmintic, tonic and choleretic. Experimentally, this plant has been shown to be devoid of antitumor activity, but does show antiviral, antibacterial, antifungal, sedative, and hypoglycemic activity.

Activity Rating = 0,0,+5,+5

PUNICACEAE _Punica granatum_ Dried pericarp	a. For diarrhea and rectocele, decoct with _Codonopsis pilosula_, _Atractylodes macrocephala_, _Glycyrrhiza uralensis_ and ginger. b. For oxyuriasis, decocted with _Areca catechu_	_Punica granatum_ has been used as a remedy for the eradication of pinworms for centuries; extracts of the plant have also shown to be anthelmintic, and the active principle (pelletierine) has been isolated from this plant and has been used for treating oxyuriasis in many countries. A high concentration of astringent tannins in the fruit of _P. granatum_ undoubtedly accounts for the antidiarrheal activity attributed to this preparation in Chinese medicine. _Areca catechu_ is well known to contain the anthelmintic alkaloid arecoline.

Activity Rating = +5,+5

PYROLACEAE

Pyrola rotundifolia

Dried whole plant

a. For rheumatic pain, decoct alone or with *Polygonum cuspidatum*, or macerate with wine for one week.

b. For tuberculosis and hemoptysis, decoct with *Stemona sessilifolia* and drink the decoction with honey.

A number of phenolic glycosides, including arbutin, homoarbutin, and isohomoarbutin, and isohomoarbutin have been isolated from *P. rotundifolia*, but their pharmacological effects have not been assessed in laboratory animals. On the other hand, arbutin is known to have antibacterial properties, and plants containing arbutin were used extensively throughout the world as urinary antiseptics in former times. However, one recent publication has shown negative *in vitro* antibacterial, antifungal, and antiviral activities for extracts of *P. rotundifolia*. Anticancer effects for extracts of *P. rotundifolia* have been assessed in laboratory animals with conflicting positive and negative results.

See *Polygonum cuspidatum* (anti-inflammatory).

Activity Rating = +4,+4

RANUNCULACEAE

Aconitum carmichaeli Dried lateral roots.	a. For colds, rigor, vomiting and as an aperient, combine with *Zingiber officinale*, *Glycyrrhiza uralensis* and decoct. b. For rheumatoid arthritis, combine with *Cinnamomum cassia*, *Atractylodes macrocephala* and *Glycyrrhiza uralensis* and decoct. c. For chest pains, stomach ache, anorexia, and as an aperient, combine with *Cinnamomum cassia*, *Zingiber officinale* and *Atractylodes macrocephala* and decoct. d. For nephritis, edema and oligouria, combine with *Cinnamomum casssia*, *Zingiber officinale*, *Atractylodes macrocephala* and *Astragalus membranaceus* and decoct.	All *Aconitum* species are highly toxic due to the cardiotoxic alkaloid aconitine, as well as perhaps others. Various *Aconitum* species have shown antitumor activity in laboratory animals. Other *Aconitum* species have shown *in vitro* antibacterial, antiviral and antifungal activity. Extracts of various *Aconitum* species have antipyretic activity. See *Glycyrrhiza uralensis* (anti-inflammatory). See *Astragalus membranaceus* (antibacterial).
Activity Rating = 0,+5,0,+5		
Anemone hupehensis var. *japonica* Whole Plant	a. For *tinea* infections, triturate the fresh leaves and use externally. b. For scrofula and dysentery, decoct and take orally.	Practically every species of *Anemone* tested to date shows antibacterial and/or antifungal activity, and the active agent is known to be the simple lactone protoanemonine. Extracts of *Anemone chinense* are also active agains *Endameba histolytica*. Other pharmacological effects of *Anemone* species are as follows: sedative, hypotensive, spasmolytic, and analgesic; extracts of these species are recognized as being vesicant, the vesicant principle being either anemonine or protoanemonine.
Activity Rating = +4,0		

Cimicifuga foetida Dried rhizome	a. For symptoms of measles, combine with Pueraria pseudo-hirsuta, Glycyrrhiza uralensis and Arctium lappa and decoct. b. For "vicious headaches" and diarrhea, combine with Nelumbo nucifera and Atractylodes lancea and decoct. c. For headache, combine with Angelica dahurica, calcium sulfate, Pueraria pseudo-hirsuta, and then decoct. d. For rectocele and prolapse of the uterus, combine with Codonopsis pilosula, Angelica sinensis and Bupleurum scorzoneraefolium and decoct.	No pharmacologic studies or folkloric uses could be found concerning Cimicifuga foetida. However, Cimicifuga dahurica has shown sedative and hypotensive effects. Other pharmacological effects for Cimicifuga species include anticancer, estrogenic, contraceptive, and in vitro antifungal and antiviral activities. Various Cimicifuga species have been used as herbal remedies outside of China as diuretics, for arthritis, female disorders, cough, stomach ailments, cancer and for fevers.
Activity Rating = 0,0,0,0		
Clematis chinensis Dried roots	a. For rheumatism, lumbago, backache and arthritis, decoct alone and mix with wine or decoct with Angelica pubescens, Angelica sinensis and Viscum coloratum. b. For bones from food which stick in the throat, decoct alone and then mix with a little vinegar and swallow it slowly.	Only two references have been found concerning C. chinensis; one concerns its use as a folkloric anticancer remedy outside of China, and the other that extracts of this plant show anticancer activity in laboratory animals. Biological effects for extracts of other Clematis species are as follows: antifungal, antibacterial, anticonvulsant, antiviral and antitumor. Other species have been used as folkloric remedies outside of China as analgesics, sedatives, and for arthritis.

		Viscum coloratum, an ingredient of the polyprescription (a) for arthritis, rheumatism, etc. could be responsible for this activity since several triterpenes from Viscum album have shown anti-inflammatory activity in animals, and these triterpenes would be expected to be present in V. coloratum.
Activity Rating = +4, +5, 0		
Clematis montana Dried stems	a. For polyuria, dysuria and strangury, combine with Plantago asiatica, Poria cocos and Polygonum aviculare and decoct. b. For edema, combine with Grifola umbellata, Alisma plantago-aquatica, and Morus alba and decoct. c. For insomnia and restlessness, combine with Rehmannia glutinosa, Lophatherum gracile and Glycyrrhiza uralensis and decoct.	Nothing of value concerning the chemical constituents or pharmacological effects of Clematis mantana could be found in the literature. See also Clematis chinensis.
Activity Rating = 0,0,+4		
Coptis chinensis Dried tuber	a. For fever, combine with Scutellaria baicalensis, Gardenia jasminoides and dococt. b. For vomiting, combine with Citrus spp., Perilla frutescens, Pinellia ternata and decoct. c. For epistaxis, and vomiting of blood, combine with Scutellaria baicalensis, and Rheum tanguticum and decoct. d. For diarrhea, combine with Saussurea lappa and grind to a	Extracts of Coptis chinensis exhibit in vitro antibacterial activity, and the active principle has been shown to be berberine. Other alkaloids present in this species are worenine, jatrorrhizine, coptisine, palmatine and columbamine. The palmatine is probably responsible for the analgesic activity attrubuted to this plant. See also reference to the antidiarrheal and antibacterial effects

		of berberine under Berberis amurensis (Berberidaceae). See Pinellia ternata (antiemetic).

Activity Rating = +2,+5,0,+5,+5

Pulsatilla chinensis Dried root	a. For diarrhea, amebiasis and bloody stools, decoct with Coptis chinesis, Phellodendron amurense and Fraxinus rhynchophylla	Nothing of value was found in the literature with regard to the chemical constituents or pharmacological activities of Pulsatilla chinensis. However, the prescription for diarrhea would be effective on the basis of the berberine content in Coptis chinensis. See Coptis chinensis and Berberis amurensis for further details.

Activity Rating = 5

Ranunculus zuccarinii Dried tuber	a. For swelling, combine with Paris polyphylla and Semiaquilegia adoxoides.	Nothing of value was found in the literature relative to the chemical constituents ans pharmacological activities of Ranunculus zuccarinii. However, protoanemonine is present in virtually all Ranunculus species, and is the agent responsible for most Ranunculus species. Indeed, two Ranunculus species (R. acris and R. glaber) have shown antitumor activity in animals. Protoanemonine, a lactonic compound, would be predicted to elicit this effect. If "swellings" could be interpreted as a type of tumor or other malignant growth, then the prescription indicated could well

		have a scientific basis for use. Also, *Paris polyphylla* has been reported to have antitumor activity in animals, thus further justifying the use of this prescription in Traditional Chinese medicine.
Activity Rating = +5		
Semiaquilegia adoxoides Root	a. Dococt alone as an anti-inflammatory, diuretic and antitoxic. b. Use as a tincture for dermatitis and inflammation, taken orally. c. For mastitis and dermatitis, as well as for insect and snake bites, grind the fresh root and apply externally as a paste. d. For oligouria from venereal disease, decoct and take by mouth or decoct with *Polygonum aviculare* and *Plantago asiatica*.	*Semiaquilegia adoxoides* has been used as an herbal remedy outside of China as an antibiotic.
Activity Rating = 0,+3,0,0		

RHAMNACEAE

Zizyphus jujuba var. *spinosa*

(Syn. *Zizyphus mauritiana*)

Dried ripe seed

a. For anxiety and insomnia, decoct alone or with *Glycyrrhiza uralensis*, *Ligusticum wallichii*, *Anemarrhena asphodeloides* and *Poria cocos*.
b. For hand and foot fever, night sweats and dizziness, decoct with *Paeonia lactiflora*, *Schisandra chinensis* and *Ostrea* spp.

Zizyphus jujuba has been used as a herbal remedy outside of China for the following: epilepsy, analgesic, stomach disorders, laxative, diuretic, for fevers, wound healing, as an antibiotic, and for cancer. Other *Zizyphus* species have been used as herbal remedies as sedatives, for stomach ailments, for snake bite, and as laxatives, for malaria, as analgesics, hemostatics, rheumatism, wound healing and as antibiotics. No chemical or pharmacological activity data of interest could be found on *Zizyphus jujuba*, however, *Zizyphus abyssinica* extracts have shown sedative activity in animals, as well as hypotensive, cardiotonic and smooth muscle relaxing properties. With respect to prescription (b), paeoniflorin, which would be predicted bo be present in *Paeonia lactiflora*, has been shown to elicit antipyretic properties.

Activity Rating = +4,+4

ROSACEAE

Agrimonia viscidula Dried aboveground parts	a. For vomiting of blood, decoct alone, or with *Nelumbo nucifera* and *Thuja orientalis*. b. For dysentery and bloody stools, decoct with *Sophora japonica*, *Sanguisorba officinalis* and *Schizonepeta tenuifolia*. c. From exhaustion due to overwork, decoct with *Zizyphus jujuba* fruits and take orally.	Nothing of value regarding the chemical constituents or pharmacological effects of *Agrimonia viscidula* could be found in the literature, however, several other Agrimonia species have been shown to elicit antibacterial and antifungal effects in vitro. In addition, tannins are universally present in *Agrimonia* species, which could account for their effectiveness in treating diarrhea through an astringent effect. Other *Agrimonia* species have been shown to elicit *in vivo* and *in vitro* **antiviral activity. *Agrimonia gryposepala* has shown antitumor effects in animals, undoubtedly due to the tannin content.**
Activity Rating = 0,+5,0		
Chaenomeles lagenaria Dried ripe fruit	a. For joint pains, use a tincture alone or decoct with *Stephania tetrandra*, *Clematis chinensis* and *Angelica sinensis*. b. For celialgia, diarrhea, and muscle spasms, decoct or cook with wine alone or decoct with *Agastache rugosa*, *Perilla frutescens* and *Evodia rutaecarpa*. c. For *tabes mesenterica* in children and for diarrhea, decoct alone.	Extracts of this plant have a folkloric application outside of China to treat various kidney diseases. Nothing of chemical or pharmacological interest could be found in the literature relative to this genus of plants. See *Stephania tetranda* (analgesic)
Activity Rating = +5,0,0,0		

Chaenomeles sinensis Dried ripe fruit Activity Rating = +5,0,0,0	a. Same uses as for C. lagenaria.	Same comments as for C. lagenaria.
Crataegus cuneata Dried ripe fruit Activity Rating = +4,+5	a. Same uses as Crataegus pinnatifida.	Various species of Crataegus are used clinically in Germany and Austria for increasing cardiac metabolism, coronary flow, and to some extent peripheral flow, and also for lowering blood pressure. Extracts of many species also have antiarrhythmic activity. See also Crataegus pinnatifida.
Crataegus pinnatifida Dried ripe fruit.	a. For diarrhea, combine with charcoal and then grind to a powder and add sugar. Take orally. Can also be combined with Gallus gallus domesticus, add wine and yeast and decoct. b. For stomach ache after parturition, combine with charcoal and then grind to a powder and take orally, or combine with Angelica sinensis, Leonurus heterophyllus and Zingiber officinale and decoct.	Nothing was found of interest concerning the chemical constituents or pharmacological activities of Crataegus pinnatifida. However, several other Crataegus species have common chemical constituents and pharmacological effects. All Crataegus species examined to date appear to stimulate coronary blood flow, in animals as well as in man. Extracts have an inhibitory effect on the uterus of animals. A leucoanthocyanin isolated from Crataegus oxyacantha showed sedative activity in mice. Extracts of Crataegus also show hypotensive activity in animals and in man. Tannins are universally present in Crataegus species, and

they could account for the alleged usefulness of Crataegus pinnatifida as an antidiarrheal, due to an astringent effect.

See also Crataegus cuneata.
See also Angelea sinensis (smooth muscle relaxant).

Activity Rating = +5,+5

Eriobotrya japonica Dried leaf	a. Antitussive and expectorant, decoct alone, take with honey or decoct with Platycodon grandiflorum, Prunus armeniaca, Morus alba and Peucedanum praeruptorum. b. For stomach ache, nausea, vomiting, and thirst, decoct with Pinellia ternata, Phragmites communis and Imperata cylindrica.	Nothing of interest in the literature regarding the pharmacological properties of Eriobotrya species. In prescription (a), platycodin from Platycodon grandiflorum has shown antitussive properties in animals. See Pinellia ternata (antiemetic).

Active Rating = 0,+5,+5

Prunus armeniaca Dried ripe kernel	a. For the common cold, coughs and asthma, decoct with Ephedra sinica and Glycyrrhiza uralensis. b. For constipation in old men and following childbirth in women, decoct or grind with Prunus persica, Cannabis sativa, Angelica sinensis and Citrus spp.	Prunus armeniaca has been used as an herbal remedy for cancer. No other chemical or pharmacological data regarding this species could be found in the literature. However, other Prunus species contain many pharmacologically active compounds. For example, Prunus africana extracts have yielded a steroid mixture that has been used for the treatment of prostatic hypertrophy and a patent has been issued for this use. Prunus americana extracts have shown

anticancer activity in laboratory animals. *Prunus amygdalis* has yielded an uncharacterized substance that is highly active against *Pseudomonas aeruginosa in vitro*, and against *Staphylococcus aureus* to a lesser extent. An extract of *Prunus avium*, consisting chiefly of flavonoids, was found to reversibly abolish the activity of rat and guinea pig uterus and to counteract oxytocin-induced contractions. Similar results were obtained on the rat ileum, as well as the guinea pig intestine. A similar extract of *Prunus avium* exhibited a positive inotropic effect on frog hearts damaged by quinine and posterior pituitary extract. The extract also decreased coronary resistance by 30% or more in the Langendorff rat heart preparation. Blood pressure was decreased about 10 per cent by high coronary heart flow and heart muscle contractions. It was concluded that the extract was acting via a coronary vasodilator effect. *Prunus avium* also contains pectins which could account for its value as a cough remedy. *Prunus emarginata* extracts have shown antifertility activity in experimental animals. An aqueous extract of *Prunus laurocerasus* showed analgesic and antispasmodic activities, and the volatile oil from this plant

Activity Rating = +5,0		exhibited *in vitro* antifungal activity. *Prunus lusitanica* has also shown *in vitro* antibacterial and antifungal activity, as have extracts of *Prunus padus*. *Prunus serotina* extracts have shown anticancer activity in animals. Flavonoid fractions from *Prunus spinosa* were nontoxic and caused a positive inotropic action on isolated hearts of frogs, and also demonstrated spasmolytic activity. Kaempferol from this plant showed diuretic and natriuretic action in rats. Kaempferol-3,7-dirhamnoside, isolated from *Prunus spinosa,* increased capillary resistance in animals and also was shown to have anti-inflammatory activity. Extracts of *Prunus spinosa* have been used clinically as a treatment for diarrhea, and were shown to have antibacterial activity. *Prunus virginiana* extracts have shown anticancer activity in animals. See also *Prunus mume*. See also *Ephedra sinica* (asthma) See also *Glycyrrhiza uralensis* (antitussive)
Prunus armeniaca var. *ansu* Dried ripe kernel Activity Rating = +5,0	a. The same uses as for *Prunus armeniaca*.	See also *Prunus armeniaca*, *P. mume* and *P. persica*.

Prunus mume

Dried unripe fruit

a. For chronic diarrhea and rectocele, decoct with Saussurea lappa and Nelumbo nucifera.
b. For roundworm infections, decot with Asarum heterotropoides, Zanthoxylum seed, Zingiber officinale, Coptis chinensis and Angelica sinensis, or grind the above mixture and make pills with the aide of honey.
c. As an antitussive, used as troches, or mixed with other antitussive agents.

Extracts of Prunus mume have shown activity against Mycobacterium tuberculosis in vitro and the activity was associated with the nonvolatile organic acid fraction of the plant. Prunus mume is one of several ingredients in a patented anti-narcoctic remedy containing also Scutellaria baicalensis, Citrus trifoliata, Asarum sieboldii, Tulipa edulis, Hyoscyamus niger, Taraxacum sp. Crataegus cuneata, Corydalis ambigua, Zingiber officinale, and Panax ginseng. Other pharmacologic effects for related Prunus species are noted under Prunus armeniaca.

Acting Rating = +4,0,+5

Prunus persica

Part used (?)

a. For amenorrhea due to blood clots as well as for dysmenorrhea, decoct with Angelica sinensis, Paeonia lactiflora, Ligusticum wallichii and Carthamus tinctorius.
b. For internal hemorrhages, decoct with Eupolyphaga sinensis, Ligusticum wallichii, Angelica sinensis and Typha latifolia.
c. For appendicitis, decoct with Rheum tanguticum, Paeonia suffruticosa, and watermelon seed.
d. For constipation, decot with Rheum tanguticum and Angelica sinensis and eat with honey.

For pharmacological activities of other Prunus species, see Prunus armeniaca and Prunus mume. Prescription (d) would be effective due to its content of Rheum tanguticum, which contains the known catharatic anthraquinone emodin.

See Angelica sinensis (hemostatic).

Activity Rating = +5,+5,+5,+5

Rosa laevigata Dried ripe fruit Activity Rating = 0,0,+5	a. For premature ejaculations, decoct alone or boil with sugar to make a syrup and take orally. b. For enuresis and polyuria, decoct with dried egg shell of *Hierodula* spp., the stamen of *Nelumbo nucifera* and *Dioscorea batatas*. c. For diarrhea, decoct with *Poria cocos*, *Condonopsis pilosula*, *Atractylodes macrocephala* and *Nelumbo nucifera*.	Many unidentified *Rosa* species have been used as herbal remedies for diarrhea, undoubtedly due to their tannin content which would act by an astringent mechanism. *Rosa abyssinica* extracts have shown antitumor activity in animals due to their tannin content.
Sanguisorba officinalis Dried rhizome Activity Rating = +5,+5,0	a. For bloody feces or diarrhea with blood, decoct alone and take orally, or decoct with *Glycyrrhiza uralensis*; *Agrimonia viscidula*, *Paeonia lactiflora* and *Coptis chinensis*. b. For excessive bleeding after labor, decoct with *Cyperus rotundus* and *Nelumbo nucifera*. c. For furunculosis, inflammations and burns, grind the powder and use externally or prepare a decoction and use externally.	The activity of prescription (a) can be explained on the basis of the berberine content of *Coptis chinensis*. See under *Coptis chinensis* and *Berberis amurensis*. Berberine is also a hemostatic.

RUBIACEAE

Gardenia jasminoides Dried ripe fruit	a. For jaundice and fever, combine with Artemisia capillaris, Phellodendron amurense, Rheum tanguticum, and decoct. b. For epistaxis and vomiting of blood, combine with Imperata cylindrica and decoct. c. For inflammation, grind and mix with flour, albumen and wine. Use externally.	No work has been found suggesting that G. jasminoides has antipyretic properties, however, the following Gardenia species are reported useful as antipyretics in Africa: G. abbeokutae, G. crenata, G. jovis-tonantis, G. manganjae, G. norae, G. turgida and G. radicans (folklore). Gardenia jasminoides has not been reported to elicit an effect on the liver (jaundice), but G. florida has shown choleretic activity, and the active choleretic principle has been shown to be the glycoside crocin. Interestingly enough, crocin has also been isolated from G. jasminoides, a plant used in China for treating jaundice. Gardenia jasminoides is used as an anti-inflammatory in Japan, and it has been shown experimentally to have wound healing effects. See Rheum tanguticum (choleretic).
Activity Rating = +4,0		
Knoxia corymbosa Dried tuberous root	a. For tympanites and dropsy of the abdomen as well as for constipation, decoct with Ipomoea hederacea, Saussurea lappa and hog kidney. b. For edema, grind with Euphorbia kansui and take orally.	The only reports concerning K. corymbosa are that it is a folkloric anticancer remedy, and it has yielded triterpenes, sterols and unidentified alkaloids.

	c. For skin infections, triturate with water and use externally.	
Activity Rating = 0,0		
Morinda officinalis Dried root	a. For premature ejaculations and impotence, combine with *Rehmannia glutinosa*, *Cornus officinalis* and *Rosa laevigata* and decoct. b. For polyuria and enuresis, combine with *Cornus officinalis*, *Cuscuta chinensis* and *Hierodula* sp. and decoct or grind to a powder and take orally. c. For lumbago, notalgia and weakness, combine with *Psoralea corylifolia*, *Dipsacus asper* and *Juglans sinensis* and decoct or grind to a powder and take orally. d. For cholecystitis and hernia, combine with *Foeniculum vulgare* and take orally.	*Morinda officinalis* has been used as an herbal remedy for cancer. No other information of value could be found in the literature relative to the chemical constituents and pharmacological activities of *Morinda officinalis* that would aid in substantiating the use of this plant in Traditional Chinese medicine. See *Cornus officinalis* (urinary antiseptics, antibacterial). See *Dipsacus asper* (anti-inflammatory).
Activity Rating = 0,+5,+5,0		
Rubia cordifolia Dried root	a. For epistaxis, vomiting of blood, hemoptysis and menorrhagia, decoct with charcoal or decoct with *Artemisia argyri*, *Thujax orientalis* and *Rehmannia glutinosa*. b. For amenorrhia, decoct with *Angelica sinensis* and take with wine. c. For rheumatoid arthritis, macerate the dried root with wine and seal the bottle for 10 days. Other antirheumatic drugs may also be added.	Extracts of *Rubia cordifolia* have shown *in vitro* antibacterial activity.
Activity Rating = 0,0,0		

✓ <u>Uncaria rhynchophylla</u> Dried stems and twigs Activity Rating = 0,0	a. For "liver fire" and fever, headache, dizziness and flushed face and eyes. Decoct with <u>Morus alba</u>, <u>Prunella vulgaris</u> and <u>Chrysanthemum morifolium</u>. b. For pediatric fever, colds and convulsions, decoct with <u>Lonicera japonica</u>, <u>Mentha arvensis</u>, <u>Chrysanthemum morifolium</u> and <u>Allolobophora caliginosa</u>.	<u>Uncaria rhynchophylla</u> is known to contain several hypotensive indole alkaloids.

RUTACEAE

Citrus aurantium Ripe and unripe fruit	a. For spleen and stomach ailments, chest congestion, abdominal pain and diarrhea, decoct with Atractylodes macrocephala, Coptis chinensis and Scutellaria baicalensis. b. For diarrhea and abdominal pain, decoct with Rheum tanguticum, Paeonia lactiflora and Magnolia officinalis. c. For rib pain, decoct with Bupleurum scorzoneraeflorium, Paeonia lactiflora and Glycyrrhiza uralensis. d. For rectocele caused by diarrhea and for prolapse of the uterus, decoct with Codonopsis pilosula, Astragalus membranaceus, Cimicifuga foetida and Glycyrrhiza uralensis.	Most Citrus flavonoids are well known to elicit anti-inflammatory, antibacterial and antifungal activity. Some of them show antitumor and/or cytotoxic activity in animals or in cell culture. Pectins from citrus fruits also show antibacterial and antifungal activity. Certain flavonoids from Citrus species show choleretic activity, i.e. rutoside, triethylrutoside, and quercitroside. Umbelliferone, present in virtually all Citrus species, has shown antifungal activity. Citrus aurantium has been used as an herbal remedy for high blood pressure, cancer, for allergies, as a sedative, analgesic, antispasmodic, for female disorders and as antidiarrheals. Essential oil from Citrus aurantium has shown antibacterial and antifungal activity, and three flavonoids from this plant are antifungal agents, i.e. nobiletin, tageretin and 5-hydroxy-7,8,3',4'-pentamethoxyflavone. A pyrone, named citrantin, has been isolated from Citrus aurantium and has shown antifertility activity.

Activity Rating = +5,+4,+4,0

Citrus spp. Pericarp and seed	a. For the common cold and for coughs, decoct the pericarp with	See Citrus aurantium.

Perilla frutescens, Peucedanum praeruptorum and Prunus armeniaca.
b. For coughs and excessive sputum, for nausea and vomiting, decoct the pericarp with Pinellia ternata and Poria cocos.
c. For vomiting, chest congestion and anorexia, decoct the pericarp with Zingiber officinale, Inula japonica and Pinellia ternata.
d. For coughs and chest pain, decoct with Perilla frutescens, Prunus armeniaca and Citrus aurantium.
e. For hernia, and pain in the testicles, decoct the seed with Evodia rutaecarpa, Melia toosendan, Corydalis bulbosa, Cinnamomum cassia and Citrus aurantium.

Activity Rating = +4,0,0,0,+5

Evodia rutaecarpa

Dried ripe fruit

a. For stomach chills and pain and for vomiting, take alone in a powdered form.
b. For swollen testicles, for cold and pain, decoct with Melia toosendan, Foeniculum vulgare and Citrus sp.
c. For cold and abdominal pain due to the ingestion of raw food, for vomiting and diarrhea, decoct with Saussurea lappa and Cinnamomum cassia.

Extracts of E.rutaecarpa have been used in other countries as an anti-emetic. Similar extracts have also shown antiviral activity in vitro. Various types of coumarins are widespread in the genus Evodia, and many of these have been shown to elicit significant anti-inflammatory effects in animals; thus the expected presence of coumarins in E.rutaecarpa could explain its use in reducing testicular swelling.

Activity Rating = +3,+4,+3

Phellodendron amurense

Dried bark

a. For dysentery, decoct with Pulsatilla chinensis, Fraxinus rhynchophylla and Coptis chinensis.
b. For weakness, night sweating, hematuria, lumbago, tinnitus aurium and "emissions," decoct with Rehmannia glutinosa, Anemarrhena asphodeloides and Chinemys reevesii, or remove the latter material and add Dioscorea batatas and Cornus officinalis.
c. For jaundice, decoct with Artemisia capillaris, Gardenia jasminoides and Rheum tanguticum.
d. For leucorrhea and vaginal itching, decoct with Plantago asiatica, Dioscorea batatas and Ginkgo biloba.
e. For eczema and dermatitis, decoct alone or mix with tea or oil for external use, or decoct with Sophora flavescens.

Extracts of P. amurense have shown the following biological activities in laboratory animals: choleretic, uterine stimulant, hypoglycemic, diuretic and smooth muscle relaxant. In addition, extracts have shown insecticidal activity and in vitro antiviral and antibacterial activity. Phellodendron amurense has been used as an antidiabetic remedy in China. An unidentified lactone from P. amurense has been shown to be responsible for the hypoglycemic activity, and it also lowers blood pressure, depresses the heart and stimulates rabbit intestine. A number of alkaloids have been isolated from the bark of P. amurense, including berberine, palmatine, jatrorrhizine, magnoflorine, phellodendrine and candiene. Berberine has been shown to have antibacterial activity, is useful in dysentery in humans, is a vasoconstrictor and stimulates uterine contractions. In prescription (b), the anti-inflammatory effects could be due to the diosgenin glycosides in Dioscorea batatas.

See Anemarrhena asphodeloides (anti-inflammatory).
See Dioscorea batatas (anti-inflammatory).

Activity Rating = +5,+5,+5,+5,0,+5

SAURURACEAE

Houttuynia cordata Dried whole plant	a. For chest pains, decoct and combine with Ajuga decumbens. b. For whooping cough, decoct and combine with honey or combine with Centipeda minima and decoct with water and then add honey. c. For hemorrhoids, decoct with water and use externally. d. For laryngopharyngitis, dysentery enteritis, gastritis, cough and snakebite, decoct alone.	Houttuynia cordata extracts have been used in humans for their anti-bacterial effects. This antibacterial activity has been shown to be due to compound $CH_3(CH_2)_8-(C{=}O)-CH_2-CHO$, which was isolated from the volatile oil from the seeds. This compound is very unstable in the free state, forming an inactive polymer. In addition, quercitrin was found to be the diuretic principle of this plant. See Ajuga decumbens (analgesic) See Centipeda minima (smooth muscle relaxant).

Activity Rating = +4,+5,0,+5

SAXIFRAGACEAE

Dichroa febrifuga Dried roots	a. For malaria, decoct with *Anemarrhena asphodeloides*, *Areca catechu*, *Prunus mume*, and *Zingiber officinale*.	Febrifugine (beta-dichroine) (I), the major alkaloid of *D.febrifuga*, is known to have antimalarial properties against *Plasmodium gallinaceum* in chicks. Two additional alkaloids are present in this plant, alpha-dichroine (II) and gammadichroine (III). III is 100 times more potent than quinine as an anti-malarial, II is 50 times more potent, and I is equivalent in potency to quinine.

Activity Rating = +5

SCHISANDRACEAE

Schisandra chinensis Dried ripe fruit Activity Rating = +5,0,0,+5	a. For coughs and asthma, decoct with Dioscorea batatas, Rehmannia glutinosa and Cornus officinalis. b. For premature ejaculations and night sweating, decoct with Ostrea spp., Rosa laevigata and Hierodula spp. c. For long-lasting dysentery, decoct with Evodia rutaecarpa and Psoralea corylifera. d. For insomnia, decoct with Lamprotula leai and Acorus gramineus.	Schisandra chinensis has been used as an antiseptic in folkloric medicine. Experimentally, extracts of this plant have shown in vitro activity against Mycobacterium tuberculosis. In man, the administration of an alcoholic extract of the fruit of Schisandra chinensis induced a vasodilation in the thumb which persisted for about 30 minutes. Extracts of this plant are also able to induce non-specific resistance in man, comparable to similar effects well established for Panax ginseng and Eleutherococcus senticosus in Japan, Korea and the U.S.S.R. Extracts of Schisandra chinensis also have been shown to induce hypoglycemia in animals. See also Dioscorea batatas (antitussive). See Acorus gramineus (sedative).
Schisandra sphenanthera Dried ripe fruit Activity Rating = +5,0,0,+5	a. Same uses as for Schisandra chinensis, but not as effective.	See also Schisandra chinensis.

SCROPHULARIACEAE

Rehmannia glutinosa f. *hueichingensis* Dried or fresh rhizome	a. For fever, vomiting of blood, and for bleeding, decoct with *Paeonia lactiflora*, *Paeonia suffruticosa*, *Lithospermum erythrorhizon* and *Scrophularia ningpoensis*. b. For mouth ulcers and "reddish-yellow urine," decoct with *Lophatherum gracile*, *Hocquartia manshuriensis* and fresh *Glycyrrhiza uralensis*. c. For anemia and menoxia, decoct with *Paeonia lactiflora*, *Angelica sinensis* and *Ligusticum wallichii*. d. For weak liver or kidney, lumbago, premature ejaculations, vertigo and *tinnitis aurium*, decoct with *Cornus officinalis*, *Dioscorea batatas*, *Poria cocos* and *Alisma plantago-aquatica* var. *orientale*.	Extracts of *Rehmannia lutea* have been shown to decrease blood sugar levels in laboratory animals. See *Paeonia suffruticosa* (antipyretic). See *Dioscorea batatas* (anti-inflammatory).

Activity Rating = +5,0,0,0

Scrophularia ningpoensis Dried root	a. For acute fever, sore throat and anxiety, decoct with *Lonicera japonica*, *Forsythia suspensa*, *Mentha arvensis* and *Glycyrrhiza uralensis*. b. For vomiting of blood, epistaxis and rash, decoct with *Rehmannia glutinosa* and *Paeonia suffruticosa*. c. For the late period of fever, constipation and dry throat, decoct with *Rehmannia glutinosa* and *Ophiopogon japonicus*. d. For scrofula, decoct with *Prunella vulgaris* and *Ostrea* spp.	Nothing of value was found concerning the chemical constituents or pharmacological activities of *Scrophularia ningpoensis*. See *Glycyrrhiza uralensis* (anti-inflammatory).

Activity Rating = +5,0,0,0

SELAGINELLACEAE

Selaginella tamarascina Dried whole plant	a. Use the raw material as an anticoagulant and the cooked material as a coagulant. b. For amenorrhea, decoct alone and take orally, or decoct with *Angelica sinensis*, *Paeonia lactiflora* (roots with epidermis), *Prunus persica* and *Carthamus tinctorius*. c. For bloody stools, internal hemorrhoidal bleeding and uterine bleeding, grind with *Sanguisorba officinalis*, the leaf of *Thuja orientalis*, *Schizonepeta tenuifolia* and the flower of *Sophora japonica*. d. For rectocele, use alone orally.	Nothing of value was found in the literature regarding the chemical constituents or pharmacological activities of *Selaginella tamarascina*.

Activity Rating = 0,0,0,0,0

SIMAROUBACEAE

Ailanthus altissima (Syn. Ailanthus glandulosa) Root bark and fruit	a. For dysentery, decoct the root bark alone or decoct it with Coptis chinensis, Magnolia officinalis, Saussurea lappa and Angelica sinensis. b. For leucorrhea, grind the root bark with talc and take orally, or decoct it with Sophora flavescens and Phellodendron amurense. c. For bloody stools caused by "enteric diarrhea cold", grind the fruit and eat the powder with rice soup.	Ailanthus altissima extracts have shown in vitro antibacterial activity, and they contain simaroudolides which have been shown to be effective antiprotozoan agents. In addition, when used for dysentery, it is known that Coptis chinensis contains berberine which has antibacterial activity and has shown clinical efficacy in the treatment of diarrhea in humans.
Activity Rating = +5,+5,0		
*Brucea javanica Dried ripe fruit	a. For amebic dysentery and malaria, take the seed orally. b. For condylomata acuminata and for warts, triturate the seeds into a paste and apply externally. c. For corns, or warts, use externally.	Extracts of Brucea javanica are active against cultures of Endameba histolytica and are also effective in treating amebic dysentery in humans. The effects are variously described as ranging from very effective with little toxicity, to fleeting results with relapses being common. In man and animals, gastric irritation has been described, indicated by nausea and vomiting. The viscera and other tissues showed no demonstrable pathological changes. An uncharacterized glycoside has been stated to be the active principle. Extracts of the seeds of this plant are also effective in treating malaria. Several simaroubolides have been isolated from B. javanica, and their

structures have been determined. These compounds are most likely the active antiamebic principles, but this has not yet been shown conclusively. A fixed oil from the seeds of *B. javanica* has been used for the treatment of common warts, juvenile warts and *condylomata acuminata* in humans with satisfactory results. Two related species, *B. antidysenterica* and *B. sumatrana* also contain simaroubolides and *B. sumatrana* has shown effectiveness in treating amebic dysentery, and bruceantin, bruceantarin and bruceine B from *B. antidysenterica* have shown interesting antitumor properties in animals and are cytotoxic. Thus, it is concluded that the uses for *B. javanica* in Chinese medicine are well justified.

Activity Rating = +5,+5,+5

SOLANACEAE

**Datura metel* Dried flowers	a. For asthma, combine with tobacco and make a cigarette for smoking. b. For numbmess and myalgia, prepare a decoction and use externally.	The alkaloids atropine, hyoscyamine, and scopolamine are present in all parts of *D. metel*, and they are known to act as bronchodilators when inhaled with smoke, and are also analgesic when applied locally.
Activity Rating = +5,+5		
**Hyoscyamus niger* Dried ripe seed	a. For myalgia, combine with *Glycyrrhiza uralensis* and the dried dung of *Trogopterus uralensis* and decoct. b. For coughs and asthma, combine with *Citrus* spp. and the seed of *Perilla frutescens* and decoct. c. For epilepsy, combine with *Rheum tanguticum*, *Angelica sinensis*, *Magnolia officinalis* and the fruit of *Citrus aurantium* and decoct. d. For toothache, combine with *Rehmannia glutinosa* and decoct.	All of the medicinal uses for *Hyoscyamus niger* can be explained on the basis of the well established parasympatholytic, analgesic and antiasthmatic activities of the alkaloids atropine, hyoscyamine and scopolamine, which are constituents of this plant.
Activity Rating = +5,+5,0,+5		
Lycium barbarum Dried ripe fruit and root bark	a. For impotence and backache, decoct with *Rehmannia glutinosa* and *Viscum coloratum*. b. For dizziness, decoct with *Chrysanthemum morifolium*, *Cornus officinalis*, *Dioscorea batatas*, and *Rehmannia glutinosa*. c. For weakness and fever, decoct with *Anemarrhena asphodeloides*, *Angelica sinensis*, *Artemisia apiacea* and *Gentiana macrophylla*.	*Lycium barbarum* has been reported to give hypoglycemic effects in animals. The related *L. chinense*, which is used for the same purposes as *L. barbarum*, has shown CNS stimulant and autonomic effects in mice, hypoglycemic, hyperglycemic and antifungal effects, and has been used as an herbal remedy in China for hypertension, nephritis and for cancer.
Active Rating = 0,0,0,+3		

Lycium chinense Dried ripe fruit and root bark Activity Rating = 0,0,0,+3	Same as for L. barbarum	See comments under L. barbarum.
Physalis francheti var. bunyardii Dried calyx or whole plant Activity Rating = 0,+5,0	a. For cough, sore throat, whooping cough and acute bronchitis, grind the whole plant and eat the powder, or decoct the calyx with Arctium lappa, Scrophularia ningpoensis and Glycyrrhiza ningpoensis. b. For pemphigus, triturate the fresh plant and apply it on the infected area.	Nothing of value was found in the literature with regard to the chemical constituents or pharmacological activities of Physalis francheti.
✓Solanum nigrum (Syn. Solanum americanum) Whole plant	a. For dermatitis and inflammation, decoct alone and take orally. b. For heavy female discharges, decoct alone and take orally. c. Can be used for sore throat and diarrhea.	Solanum nigrum is considered as a poisonous plant due to the steroidal alkaloids present in it. It has been used as an herbal sedative, cardiotonic, antitussive, choleretic, antidiarrheal, diuretic and antipyretic. Extracts of Solanum nigrum show CNS depression, decrease cardiac activity, reduce blood pressure, cause vasodilation, are analgesic and have antispasmodic activity. Extracts also protect the liver of rats from experimental carbon tetrachloride toxicity, and have antibacterial activity. Solanum nigrum contains diosgenin, which shows anti-inflammatory activity in laboratory animals. Some of the Solanum

glycoalkaloids that have pharmacological activity are solanine solasonine and solamargine (antifungal) and solanocapsine (antibacterial). An extract of *Solanum tomatillo* has shown hypothermic activity in animals.

Activity rating = +5,0,+3

SPARGANIACEAE

Sparganium stoloniferum

Dried plant

Activity Rating = +5,0

a. For clots, abdominal pain, amenorrhea, decoct with Angelica sinensis, Carthamus tinctorius and Rehmannia glutinosa, or decoct with Ligusticum wallichii, Paeonia suffruticosa, Cyathula capitata and Corydalis bulbosa.
b. Can be used as an expectorant and for abdominal and chest pain.

Nothing of value was found in the literature with regard to the chemical constituents and pharmacological activities of Sparganium stoloniferum.

See Angelica sinensis (smooth muscle relaxant, anti-inflammatory). See Corydalis bulbosa (analgesic).

STEMONACEAE

Stemona sessilifolia Dried root	a. For tuberculosis, grind alone and take twice a day. b. For coughs and sore throat, decoct with *Schizonepeta tenuifolia*, *Cynanchum stauntoni* and *Platycodon grandiflorum*. c. For whooping cough, decoct alone and take with sugar or decoct with *Cynanchum stauntoni* and *Glehnia littoralis*. d. For oxyuriasis, decoct alone and use as an enema. e. For head lice, prepare a tincture and use externally.	*Stemona sessilifolia* has been shown to have antibacterial properties *in vitro*. See *Platycodon grandiflorum* (antitussive).

Activity Rating = +5,+5,0,0,0,0

TAMARICACEAE

<u>Tamarix chinensis</u> Dried young stem and leaf	a. For the symptoms of measles, decoct with <u>Cimicifuga foetida</u>, <u>Schizonepeta tenuifolia</u> and <u>Arctium lappa</u>. b. For acute fevers, decoct with <u>Mentha arvensis</u>, <u>Schizonepeta tenuifolia</u>, <u>Xanthium strumarium</u>, and use both orally and externally. c. For skin itching, decoct or grind with <u>Angelica sinensis</u> and <u>Glycyrrhiza uralensis</u>.	Nothing of value was found in the literature with regard to the chemical constituents or pharmacological activities of <u>Tamarix chinensis</u>. See <u>Glycyrrhiza uralensis</u> (anti-inflammatory).

Activity Rating = 0,0,+5

THYMELAEACEAE

Aquilaria sinensis The black-brown stem with resin.	a. For chest and abdominal pain, triturate with Lindera strychnifolia and take the filtrate orally. b. For "weakness" in old people and for asthma, decoct with Aconitum carmichaeli, Zingiber officinale, Schisandra chinensis and Cinnamomum cassia.	The only information available on Aquilaria species is that Aquilaria sinensis has been used as an herbal remedy for high blood pressure and as a choleretic, and that Aquilaria agallochum is used as an herbal remedy for cancer, and as a general tonic.

Activity Rating = 0,0

TYPHACEAE

Typha latifolia Dried pollen	a. Use alone uncooked as an anticoagulant or cooked as a coagulant. b. For blood in the urine and pain, decoct with *Abutilon avicennae*, *Rehmannia glutinosa*, *Gardenia jasminoides* and *Cephalanopsis segetum*. c. For amenorrhea and abdominal pain, and abdominal pain after labor, triturate with *Trogoterus xanthipes*, add black sugar, and use orally with water or wine. d. For vomiting of blood, decoct with *Gardenia jasminoides*, *Rehmannia glutinosa*, *Imperata cylindrica* and *Scutellaria baicalensis*. e. For internal hemorrhages, decoct with *Prunus persica*, *Ligusticum wallichii*, *Carthamus tinctorius*, and a cup of "baby stool". f. For children who "swallow their tongues," use alone in powder form, for external use.	Nothing of value was found in the literature with regard to the chemical constituents or pharmacological activities of *Typha latifolia*. See *Imperata cylindrica* (hemostatic).

Activity Rating = 0,0,0,+5,0,0

UMBELLIFERAE

Angelica anomala Root Activity Rating = 0,0,0,0,0	a. Same uses as Angelica dahurica.	See Angelica dahurica.
Angelica dahurica Dried root Activity Rating = 0,0,0,0,0	a. For the common cold and headache, grind to a powder and take alone or decoct with Ledebouriella seseloides, Ligusticum wallichii and Notopterygium incisum. b. For common cold fever and headache, decoct with Scutellaria baicalensis. c. For sinus headache, decoct with Xanthium strumarium, Mentha arvensis, Agastache rugosa and Asarum heterotropoides. d. For furunculosis, abscesses and skin itching, as well as snake bite and leucorrhea.	Angelica dahurica has not been investigated pharmacologically, but has yielded the coumarins byakangelicol, xanthotoxin and bergapten, as well as others. in addition, triterpenes and sterols are reported present in this species. The coumarins would be predicted to have anti-inflammatory properties. See also Angelica pubescens, and Angelica sinensis.
Angelica pubescens Dried rhizome and roots Activity Rating = +5,0	a. For rheumatic arthritis and lumbago, decoct with Viscum coloratum, Ledebouriella seseloides and Angelica sinensis. b. For the common cold and headaches.	Angelica pubescens has not been investigated pharmacologically, but has yielded the following coumarins: angelol, bergapten, glabra lactone and umbelliferone, as well as flavonoids and triterpenes and sterols. The coumarins would be expected to have anti-inflammatory activity. See also Angelica dahurica and Angelica sinensis. See also Viscum coloratum (anti-inflammatory).

Angelica sinensis Dried root	a. For menoxenia, decoct with Ligusticum wallichii, Paeonia lactiflora and Rehmannia glutinosa. b. For amenorrhea, decoct with the above mixture (a) and Carthamus tinctorius. c. For dysmenorrhea, decoct with (a) above and Corydalis bulbosa. d. For anemia, decoct with Astragalus membranaceus or decoct with Cinnamomum cassia, Paeonia lactiflora, Zingiber officinale, Zizyphus jujuba and maltose. e. For venous thrombosis, decoct with Angelica sinensis, Lonicera japonica, Scrophularia ningpoensis and Glycyrrhiza uralensis. f. For constipation, decoct with Cannabis sativa and honey.	Angelica sinensis has been used as a folkloric remedy for diabetes, hypertension and nephritis, as well as for cancer. Extracts of this species have shown in vitro and in vivo antiviral activity. Angelica glauca and Angelica archangelica have been used outside of China as remedies for diarrhea, and various Angelica species have shown the following pharmacological activities in animals: anticancer, photosensitization, hemostatic, CNS depressant, smooth muscle relaxant (due to volatile oil), and anti-inflammatory, as well as in vitro antibacterial, antifungal and antiviral activity. See also Angelica dahurica and Angelica pubescens. See Corydalis bulbosa (analgesic).

Activity Rating = 0,0,+5,0,+5,0

*Bupleurum scorzonerae-folium (Syn. Bupleurum falcatum) Dried root or whole plant	a. For malaria and the common cold, decoct with Scutellaria baicalensis and Pinellia ternata. b. For tympanites of the liver and abdomen, decoct with Paeonia lactiflora, Citrus aurantium and Glycyrrhiza uralensis. c. For menoxenia and dysmenorrhea, decoct with Angelica sinensis, Paeonia lactiflora and Atractylodes macrocephala. d. For prolapse of the uterus and rectocele, decoct with	Bupleurum scorzoneraefolium (B. falcatum) has been used as a folkloric remedy outside of China for the following conditions: anticancer, antipyretic and hypotensive. Experimentally, it has been shown that this plant has choleretic, antipyretic, hypoglycemic, anticancer, smooth muscle relaxant, strengthening of capillaries, anti-inflammatory, and analgesic activities. The active principles appear to be a mixture

	Cimicifuga foetida, Codonopsis pilosula and Angelica sinensis.	of triterpene glycosides, referred to as saikosides, which have been shown to have the following pharmacological effects in animals: hypotensive, cardiotonic, anti-inflammatory, antihistaminic, sedative, analgesic, antipyretic, antitussive, intestinal stimulant, and antiulcer effects. In addition, extracts of this plant have shown in vitro antibacterial and antiviral activity, the latter probably being due to a volatile oil. Other related species of Bupleurum have been shown to elicit choleretic and antipyretic effects.
Activity Rating = +5,0,+5,0		
Changium smyrnioides Dried root	a. For coughs, decoct with Morus alba, Eriobotrya japonica and Glycyrrhiza uralensis. b. For nausea and vomiting, decoct with Inula japonica, Pinellia ternata, Zingiber officinale and ferric oxide.	Nothing of value was found in the literature regarding the chemical constituents or pharmacological effects of plants in the genus Changium. See Glycyrrhiza uralensis (antitussive). See Pinellia ternata (antiemetic).
Activity Rating = +5,+5,0		
Foeniculum vulgare Dried ripe fruit	a. For hernia and lower abdominal pain, grind with Citrus sp. and add fried Crataegus pinnatifida (or C. cuneata), and eat with wine. In serious cases, decoct with Evodia rutaecarpa, Saussurea lappa and Corydalis bulbosa.	The volatile oil from F. vulgare has been investigated pharmacologically in animals and has been shown to relax smooth muscle, which could explain the effect of decoctions of this plant in dysmenorrhea. Extracts of F.

	b. For dysmenorrhea, decoct with Angelica sinensis, Paeonia lactiflora, Cyperus rotundus and Corydalis bulbosa.	vulgare are devoid of uterine stimulant activity in laboratory animals. See Corydalis bulbosa (analgesic).
Activity Rating = +5,+5,+5		
Glehnia littoralis Dried root	a. For hacking cough and thirst, combine with Ophiopogon japonicus, Polygonatum officinale, Trichosanthes kirilowii and Morus alba and decoct. b. For cough and croup, combine with Rehmannia glutinosa, Scrophularia ningpoensis, Anemarrhena asphodeloides and Arctium lappa and decoct. c. For fever and thirst, combine with Rehmannia glutinosa, Polygonatum officinale, Ophiopogon japonicus and decoct. d. For chest pain, hyperacidity, thirst, and for improving liver and kidney function, combine with Ophiopogon japonicus, Angelica sinensis, Lycium chinense, Rehmannia glutinosa and Melia toosendan and decoct.	Nothing of value was found in the literature with regard to the chemical constituents or pharmacological activities of plants in the genus Glehina.
Activity Rating = +3,0,0,+3		
Ledebouriella seseloides Dried roots	a. For the common cold, decoct with Schizonepeta tenuifolia, Perilla frutescens var. crispa and ginger. b. For migraine headaches, decoct with Angelica dahurica and Ligusticum wallichii. c. For rheumatoid arthritis, decoct with Angelica pubescens, Viscum coloratum and Gentiana macrophylla.	No data could be found on the chemical constituents or pharmacological activities of Ledebouriella seseloides, however, the additional ingredients in polyprescription (c) offer evidence that the prescriptions themselves could have the activities attributed to them.

	d. For ophthalmia, eye swelling and pain, decoct with Morus alba, Chrysanthemum morifolium and Gardenia jasminoides.	For example, gentianine is present in Gentiana macrophylla, and this alkaloid has been well documented to have anti-inflammatory properties. See also Viscum coloratum (anti-inflammatory).
Activity Rating = 0,0,+5,+3		
Ligusticum wallichii Dried rhizome	a. For anemia and menoxenia, decoct with Angelica sinensis, Paeonia lactiflora and Rehmannia glutinosa. b. For the common cold and headaches, decoct with Ledebouriella seseloides, Mentha arvensis, Schizonepeta tenufolia and Angelica dahurica. c. For dizziness, decoct with Morus alba, Uncaria rhynchophylla and Chrysanthemum morifolium.	No papers have been found that would allow one to speculate on the biological activities of Ligusticum wallichii in man.
Activity Rating = 0,0,0		
Notopterygium incisum Dried root or rhizome	a. For the common cold, headache, excessive sweating and joint pains, decoct with Ledebouriella seseloides, Angelica dahurica and Asarum heterotropoides var. mandshuricum. b. For rheumatic arthritis and lumbago, decoct with Angelica pubesens, Gentiana macrophylla and Morus alba.	Nothing of value was found in the literature regarding the chemical constituents or pharmacological activities of Notopterygium incisum. See Angelica dahurica (anti-inflammatory). See Gentiana macrophylla (anti-inflammatory).
Activity Rating = +5,+5		

Peucedanum praeruptorum Dried root Activity Rating = +5,0	a. For influenza, use as an antitussive and expectorant, decoct with Mentha arvensis, Arctium lappa, Prunus armeniaca and Platycodon grandiflorum. b. For chest pains, add Perilla frutescens, Citrus spp. and Citrus aurantium.	Nothing of value was found in the literature regarding the chemical constituents and pharmacological activities of Peucedanum species that would contribute to an understanding of the use of this plant in Traditional Chinese medicine. See Prunus armeniaca (antitussive). See Platycodon grandiflorum (antitussive).

VALERIANACEAE

Valeriana stubendorfi

Dried rhizomes and roots

a. For use as a sedative and anticonvulsant, use alone.
b. For epilepsy, decoct with *Citrus* sp.
c. For neurasthenia and insomnia, use alone.

Although nothing has been published concerning the pharmacology of *Valeriana stubendorfi*, or its chemical constituents, several related *Valeriana* species have been studied and all of them exhibit similar biological activities and yield similar chemical compounds. It is well established, for example, that *Valeriana* species are sedative in animals and in man. The active principles are iridoid valepotriates, and these are currently being marketed in Europe as sedatives. Other pharmacological effects in animals of *Valeriana* species are as follows: analgesic, hypotensive (active principle is valeric acid), anticonvulsant, tranquillizer, anti-diuretic, antipyretic, and *in vitro* extracts of *Valeriana* species have antibacterial properties. Thus, it is concluded that *V. stubendorfi* does have properties attributed to it by Chinese medicine.

Activity Rating = +4,+4,+4

VERBENACEAE

Callicarpa dichotoma Leaves	a. For internal hemorrhages, grind to powder or prepare a decoction and take orally. b. For wound healing and external hemorrhages, grind to a powder and use externally or grind the fresh leaves and use externally. c. For keratitis and snake bite.	Nothing was found concerning Callicarpa dichotoma. The following species have been used as herbal remedies outside of China: C.macrophylla as a diuretic and antibacterial, and for skin diseases and as an antibacterial; C.caudata for reheumatism; C.longifolia and C.americana for cancer; C.elegans as an analgesic and C.formosana as an insecticide. An unidentified Callicarpa species has been used in herbal medicine as a contraceptive. Callicarpa candicans (C.cana) has has shown piscicidal activity and the furanoid diterpene maingayic acid has been identified as the piscicidal constituent of Callicarpa maingayi, as has 5,6,7-trimethoxyflavone been identified as the piscicidal constituent of Callicarpa japonica.
Activity Rating = 0,+2,0		
Clerodendrum trichotomum Leaves	a. For hypertension and rheumatic pains, prepare a decoction and combine it with Siegesbeckia pubescens, decoct again or grind to a powder and mix with honey to make pills. b. For dermatitis, prepare a decoction and use externally, or combine with Houttuynia cordata and decoct. Use externally.	Extracts of C. trichotomum have shown anti-inflammatory activity in laboratory animals.
Activity Rating = +5,+5		

VITACEAE

Ampelopsis japonica Dried roots	a. For "sloughing ulcers" and dermatitis, decoct alone and take orally, or grind to a powder, add water, and apply externally. b. For burns and frostbite ulcers, grind to a powder and use externally or grind with *Phellodendron amurense* and sesame oil and apply externally. c. For leucorrhea and uterine discharge, decoct and use orally. d. For acne, triturate with *Prunus armeniaca* and egg white and apply externally.	Nothing of chemical or pharmacological interest could be found with respect to the genus *Ampelopsis*.

Activity Rating = 0,0,0,0

ZYGOPHYLLACEAE

Tribulus terrestris
(syn. Tribulus lanuginosa)

Dried ripe fruit

a. Use alone for "liver fire", and for improving the appetite.
b. For headache, dizziness and chest congestion, decoct with Chrysanthemum morifolium and Uncaria rhynchophylla.
c. For eye inflammations, decoct with Chrysanthemum morifolium, Equisetum hiemale, Celosia argentea and Cassia tora.

Tribulus terrestris has been used as an herbal remedy for the following: high blood pressure, cardiotonic, diuretic, antipyretic, aphrodisiac, antitussive, antihemorrhagic, cancer, and it is known to be a toxic plant. Experimentally, in the anesthetized dog, extracts of Tribulus terrestris fruits produced diuresis and increased the creatinine renal clearance which suggested increased glomerular filtration. The extract did not signficantly increase the chloride clearance, which excludes inhibition of tubular chloride reabsorbtion. These effects were not produced by an ether extract of the fruits. Since diosgenin, gitogenin and chlorogenin have been isolated from this plant, and these sapogenins are known to elicit anti-inflammatory effects in animals, it would be expected that extracts of Tribulus terrestris would also elicit this same effect. This plant also contains the known pharmacologically active alkaloids harman and harmine.

Activity Rating = 0,0+5

ANIMAL PRODUCTS AND NON-PLANT DRUGS USED IN TRADITIONAL CHINESE MEDICINE

Agkistrodon acutus Dried body without internal organs Activity Rating = 0	a. For rheumatoid arthritis, stroke causing paralysis, skin infections, tetanus and convulsions, grind into a powder or macerate with wine and take orally.	Nothing of value could be found in the literature regarding the chemical constituents or pharmacological effects of Agkistrodon species, other than the toxic effects of venom.
Allolobophora caliginosa Dried whole body Activity Rating = 0,0,0,0,0	a. For high fever convulsions, decoct with Buthus matensi, Uncaria rhynchophylla and Forsythia suspensa. b. For hypertension, decoct or take the ground powder alone. c. For monoplegia, decoct with Angelica sinensis, Ligusticum wallichii, Carthamus tinctorius, Paeonia lactiflora and Astragalus membranaceus. d. For dysuria, decoct alone and take orally. e. For asthma and bronchitis, decoct and take orally.	Nothing of value was found in the literature with regard to this organism.
Bombyx mori (Silkworm) Dried body and feces Activity Rating = 0,+5	a. For infant's cold, decoct with Gastrodia elata, Arisaema consanguineum, Acorus calamus and Citrus spp. b. For fever and headache, decoct with Equisetum hiemale, Schizonepeta tenuifolia, Morus alba and Glycyrrhiza uralensis. c. For cholera and abdominal pain, decoct with Chaenomeles lagenaria, Evodia rutaecarpa, Tetrapanax papyrifera, Pinellia ternata, Scutellaria baicalensis and Gardenia jasminoides. d. For scrofula, decoct alone.	Bombyx mori contains ecdysterones, which have been shown to have analgesic activity in animals and in man.

Chinemys reevsii Ventral shell (Tortoise)	For impotency, fever, vertigo, tinnitus aurium, and night sweating, decoct with Rehmannia glutinosa, Anemarrhena asphodeloides, Phellodendron amurense, or grind and make pills with spinal cord. b. For fever, inflammation, difficult breathing, and muscle spasm of limbs, decoct with Rehmannia glutinosa, Ostrea spp., Paeonia lactiflora and Ophiopogon japonicus. c. For menorrhagia, decoct with Phellodendron amurense, Paeonia lactifolora, Scutellaria baicalensis and Cyperus rotundus.	Nothing of value was found in the literature relative to this organism. See Paeonia lactiflora (anti-pyretic, anti-inflammatory).
Activity Rating = 0,+5,0		
Buthus martensi Dried body	a. For convulsions in children and tetanus, decoct with Bombyx mori, Allolobophora caliginosa and Gastrodia elata. b. For minor strokes, grind the powder and take orally. c. For tetanus, decoct with Scolopendra subspinipes and Uncaria rhynchophylla.	Nothing of value was found in the literature regarding the chemical constituents or pharmacological effects of this organism.
Activity Rating = 0,0,0		
Bos taurus domesticus (domesticated ox) Gall stones	a. For acute fever, high fever, unconsciousness and convulsions, grind to a powder and take orally, or decoct with Coptis chinensis,	Nothing could be found in the literature that would support the use of ox gall stones for the conditions indicated in Chinese

	Scutellaria baicalensis and *Gardenia jasminoides*. b. For dermatitis and sore throat.	Traditional medicine. See *Scutellaria baicalensis* (sedative).
Activity Rating = +5,0		
Cryptotympana atrata Skin	a. For the common cold, croup and rubella, combine with *Mentha arvensis* and decoct. b. For rouvax (?), combine with *Pueraria pseudo-hirsuta*, *Forsythia suspensa* and *Arctium lappa* and decoct. c. For ophthalmia, combine with *Chrysanthemum morifolium*, *Eriocaulon buergerianum* and *Equisetum hiemale* and decoct. d. For tetanus, combine with *Arisaema consanguineum*, *Gastrodia elata*, *Buthus martensi* and *Bombyx mori* and then decoct.	Nothing of value was found in the literature regarding the chemical constituents and biological effects of this organism. See *Equisetum hiemale* (antibacterial).
Activity Rating - 0,0,+5,0		
Eupolyphaga sinensis Dried body	a. For amenorrhea or dry skin and nails decoct with *Rehmannia glutinosa*, *Paeonia lactiflora*, *Rheum tanguticum* and *Scutellaria baicalensis*, or pulverize with *Prunus persica* and *Rhuem tanguticum* and take the powder with water. b. For internal hemorrhages, decoct with *Rheum tanguticum* and *Angelica sinensis* and use externally.	Nothing of value was found in the literature with regard to the chemical constituents or pharmacological effects of this organism. See *Angelica sinensis* (hemostatic).
Activity Rating = 0,0,+4		

Gallus gallus domesticus (Chicken) Dried gizzard	a. For diarrhea, combine with *Atractylodes macrocephala* and *Saussurea lappa* and decoct. b. For enuresis, combine with *Hierodula* sp. and then decoct.	Nothing could be found in the literature regarding the chemical constituents and pharmacological activities of *Gallus gallus domesticus* that would support its use in Traditional Chinese medicine.
Activity Rating = +3,0		
Gekko gecko Whole body without viscera.	a. For weakness and asthma, combine with *Panax ginseng* and take orally as a powder, or combine with *Codonopsis pilosula*, *Ophiopogon japonicus* and *Schisandra chinensis* and decoct. b. For coughs with bleeding, and asthma, combine with *Glehnia littoralis*, *Prunus armeniaca*, *Anemarrhena asphodeloides*, and *Morus alba* and decoct.	Nothing of value was found in the literature relative to the chemical constituents or biological effects of this organism. See *Codonopsis pilosula* (hematopoetic), See *Prunus armeniaca*, (antitussive).
Activity Rating = +5,+5,+4		
Haliotis diversicolor Shell	a. For dizziness, combine with *Rehmannia glutinosa*, *Paeonia lactiflora*, the ripe fruit of *Ligusticum lucidum* and *Chrysanthemum morifolium*, and decoct. b. For glaucoma and cataracts, combine with *Chrysanthemum morifolium*, *Morus alba*, *Glycyrrhiza uralensis* and *Celosia argentea*, and decoct.	Extracts of the related *Haliotis ovina* have shown antitumor activity in animals and extracts of *Haliotis rufescens* have shown antiviral activity *in vitro*.
Activity Rating = 0,+2		

Hierodula sp. Egg shell	a. For premature ejaculations, take as a powder with a solution of salt, or combine with *Schisandra chinensis* and *Rosa laevigata* and decoct. b. For polyuria and "absent-mindedness," combine with *Polygala tenuifolia*, *Acorus gramineus*, *Codonopsis pilosula*, and the ventral shell of *Chinemys reevesii* and decoct. c. For enuresis, combine with *Diosocrea batatas*, *Cuscuta chinensis* and *Schisandra chinensis*, make a powder, and decoct.	Nothing of value was found in the literature regarding the chemical constituents or biological effects of this organism.

Activity Rating = 0,0,0

Hirudo nipponica Dried body (leech) Activity Rating = 0,0,0	a. Same uses as for Whitmania pigra.	Nothing of value was found in the literature relative to the chemical constituents and pharmacological effects of this organism.
Lamprotula leai Shell Activity Rating = +3,0,+5	a. For "liver fire", dizziness, headache, tinnitus aurium, and flushed face, decoct with Polygonum multiflorum, Ligustrum lucidum and Eclipta prostrata, or decoct with Morus alba, Chrysanthemum morifolium and Prunella vulgaris. b. For palpitations and insomnia, decoct with Polygala tenuifolia, Zizyphus jujuba, Angelica sinensis and Rehmannia glutinosa.	Nothing of value was found in the literature regarding the chemical constituents or pharmacological effects of this organism. See Angelica sinensis (sedative).
Ostrea spp. (Oyster) Activity Rating = +5,+5,0,0	a. For impotence, vertigo and headache, decoct with Chinemys reevesii, Achyranthes bidentata and Paeonia lactiflora. b. For night sweating or sweating, decoct with Astragalus membranaceus, Triticum aestivum and Paeonia lactiflora. c. For premature ejaculations, decoct with Rosa laevigata. d. For scrofula, decoct with Scrophularia ningpoensis and Prunella vulgaris.	Proteins with insulin-like activity have been isolated from Ostrea edulis. Ecdysones present in Achyranthes species have shown analgesic activity in humans. See Paeonia lactiflora (antipyretic).

Scolopendra subspinipes mutilans Dried body (a centipede)	a. For tetanus and convulsions, decoct with Uncaria rhynchophylla, Bombyx mori, Buthus martensi and Allolobophora caliginosa. b. For scrofula and ulcers, use alone with tea leaf (Camellia sinensis). Grind to a powder and use externally.	Nothing of value was found in the literature regarding this organism.
Activity Rating = 0,0		
Sepia esculenta Bone (cuttlefish)	a. For peptic ulcer and lung bleeding, grind to a powder and take orally, or prepare a decoction and take orally. b. For stomachache and acid stomach, grind to a powder and take orally or mix with Fritillaria thunbergii, grind the mixture to a powder, and take orally. c. For bronchitis and asthma, grind to a powder and take orally with water. d. For heavy female discharges, grind with Angelica dahurica and Rubia cordifolia and take orally or decoct both plants and take orally. e. For menorrhagia, decoct with Rubia cordifolia and Ostrea spp.	Nothing of value was found in the literature, however, the bone would contain calcium which would act as an antacid and be a rational explanation for the use of one of the prescriptions for acidic stomach.
Activity Rating = 0,+5,0,0,0		
Trogopterus xanthipes Dried animal excretion	a. Use alone for circulation, as an anticoagulant and as an analgesic. b. For amenorrhea and abdominal pain after labor, triturate with Typha latifolia, add boiled water, black sugar and wine and take orally. c. For intestinal "cold" pain and stomach pain, triturate with Zingiber officinalis and wine and take orally.	Nothing of value was found in the literature relative to the chemical constituents and pharmacological effects of this organism.
Activity Rating = 0,0,0		

<u>Whitmania pigra</u> Dried body	a. For amenorrhea, or abdominal pain caused by blood clots, use the dried powder orally, or combine with <u>Angelica sinensis</u>, <u>Prunus persica</u>, <u>Sparganium stoloniferum</u> and <u>Leonurus heterophyllus</u>, and decoct. b. For inflammation by unknown poisons, decoct and take orally.	Nothing of value was found relative to the chemical constituents and biological effects of this organism.
Activity Rating = 0,0,0		
Sodium sulfate	a. For stomach and intestinal fever and constipation, decoct with <u>Rheum tanguticum</u>, <u>Citrus aurantium</u> and <u>Magnolia officinalis</u>.	The activity of this prescription can be rationally explained on the basis of the <u>Rheum tanguticum</u>, which contains known cathartic anthraquinones.
Activity Rating = +5		

Appendix B

MEMBERS OF THE HERBAL PHARMACOLOGY GROUP TO THE PEOPLE'S REPUBLIC OF CHINA

Louis Lasagna (Chairman)
Chairman of the Department of Pharmacology and Toxicology
University of Rochester
Rochester, New York

John J. Burns
Vice President for Research
Hoffmann-LaRoche, Inc.
Nutley, New Jersey

Norman R. Farnsworth
Head of the Department of Pharmacognosy and Pharmacology
University of Illinois at the Medical Center
Chicago, Illinois

S. Morris Kupchan
John W. Mallet Professor of Chemistry
University of Virginia
Charlottesville, Virginia

Thomas H. Maren
Chairman of the Department of Pharmacology and Therapeutics
University of Florida
Gainesville, Florida

Yvonne Chu Meinwald
Lecturer in Chemistry
Cornell University
Ithaca, New York

George R. Pettit
Professor of Chemistry
Arizona State University
Tempe, Arizona

Micharl A. Schwartz
Dean of the School of Pharmacy
State University of New York
Buffalo, New York

Patricia Jones Tsuchitani
Staff Officer
Committee on Scholarly Communication with the People's Republic of China
National Academy of Sciences
Washington, D.C.

Frederic E. Wakeman, Jr.
Chairman of the Center for Chinese Studies
University of California
Berkeley, California

E. Leong Way
Chairman of the Department of Pharmacology and Experimental Therapeutics
University of California Medical Center
San Francisco, California

Murray D. Zinoman
Bureau of Educational and Cultural Affairs/East Asia
Department of State
Washington, D.C.

Appendix C

Itinerary

June 1, 1974	Arrival in Kwangchow (Canton) by train from Hong Kong. Visit the Tung Fang Hung Kindergarten.
June 2	Sightseeing at Fo-shan: porcelain factory and ancestral temple. Depart on 6:00 PM flight to Peking.
June 3	Visit the Peking Arts and Handicraft Factory. Sightseeing at the Summer Palace.
June 4	Kuang An Men Hospital, Peking Institute of Chinese Materia Medica of the Academy of Chinese Traditional Medicine.
June 5	Peking Hospital of Chinese Traditional Medicine Visit Forbidden City and Palace Museum
June 6	Fu Wai Hospital Peking University, Department of Organic Chemistry and Biochemistry
June 7	Institute of Materia Medica of the Chinese Academy of Medical Sciences
June 8	Experimental Plantation of the Insitute of Materia Medica, Peking suburbs Jih T'an Hospital and Tumor Prevention Research Institute
June 9	Visit the Great Wall and the Ming Tombs
June 10	Travel by train to Tientsin. Visit Nan K'ai Hospital
June 11	Tientsin Hospital Return to Peking by train
June 12	Capital Hospital, Peking Seminar and lectures by members of delegation.
June 13	Travel by air to Shanghai
June 14	Shanghai Institute of Materia Medica Tsao Yang New Workers Village, in Shanghai suburb
June 15	Lung Hua Hospital of Traditional Medicine Shanghai #2 Pharmaceutical Factory of Chinese Traditional Drugs

Itinerary

June 16	Shanghai Industrial Exhibition Peng Pu People's Commune, in Shanghai suburb
June 17	Take early morning flight to Nanking. Visit Nanking Yangtze River Bridge Nanking College of Pharmacy
June 18	Kiangsu Provincial Hospital of Chinese Traditional Medicine, Nanking. Visit tomb of Sun Yat-sen outside of Nanking Take evening flight back to Shanghai
June 19	One group visits Lu Hsun Memorial One group visits Jui Chin Hospital Afternoon: everyone visits Shanghai Children's Palace
June 20	One group visits the Shanghai Third Middle School One group visits Hua Shan Hospital One group visits Shanghai Historical Museum Afternoon: one group visits site of 1st Congress of Chinese Communist Party and the Soochow Gardens. Other group visits Institute of Organic Chemistry
June 21	Travel by train to Hangchow Take boat ride on the West Lake
June 22	Visit silk factory Visit West Lake Factory of Bamboo Products
June 23	Further sightseeing in Hangchow Take noon flight to Kwangchow Visit Kwangchow Historical Museum
June 24	Kwangtung Botanical Garden, Kwangchow Kwangtung College of Chinese Traditional Medicine
June 25	Chung Shan Medical College and its affiliated hospitals
June 26	Departure by train for Hong Kong.

Appendix D

Chinese Hosts for the Herbal Pharmacology Study Group

Peking

Chung Lin 钟林
Deputy Secretary General
Chinese Medical Association

Lü Pin (Mme) 吕斌
Staff Member
Chinese Medical Association

Wu Chung-hao 吴钟浩
Staff Member and interpreter
Chinese Medical Association

Ssu-t'u Fen-sheng 司徒奋生
Staff Member and interpreter
Chinese Medical Association

(The above four persons accompanied the group throughout the visit in China)

Hao Chan-chung 郝展君
Staff Member
Chinese Medical Association

Ma Su-yün 馬素雲
Staff Member
Chinese Medical Association

Tientsin

Chang Hua-ssu 张华四
Leading Member
Tientsin Medical Association

Li Li 李力
Deputy Secretary General
Tientsin Medical Association

Shanghai

Ho Ch'iu-cheng 何秋澄
Leading Member
Shanghai Branch
Chinese Medical Association

Liu Chih-yü 刘志玉
Deputy Secretary General
Shangahi Branch
Chinese Medical Association

Pan Hao-ch'in (Mme) 潘鶴琴
Staff Member
Shanghai Branch
Chinese Medical Association

Huang Ch'in 黄沁
Associate Professor
Department of Pharmacy
Shanghai First Medical College

Sun Shih-liang 孫时良
Instructor
Department of Pharmacy
Shanghai First Medical College

Pai Tung-lu 白東魯
Deputy Chief
Research Section of Chemical Synthesis
Shanghai Institute of Materia Medica

Sun Shu-jung 孫叔荣
Head of Medicinal Plant Group
College of Chinese Traditional Medicine
Shanghai

Nanking

Chi Wen-liang 季文良
Leading Member
Kiangsu Branch
Chinese Medical Association

Ch'en I-wang 陈亦旺
Secretary General
Kiangsu Branch
Chinese Medical Association

Ch'en Ch'iung-hua 陈琼华
Professor
Nanking School of Pharmacy

Fu Chung-han 傅仲汉
Deputy Director
Kiangsu Hospital of Chinese
Traditional Medicine

Su Huai-chieh 苏怀桔
Leading Member
Kiangsu Provincial Foreign Affairs
Service Office

Lu K'un-huai 陸坤怀
Staff Member and interpreter
Kiangsu Provincial Foreign Affairs
Service Office

Hangchow

Lai Kuang-hsing 賴光兴
Leading Member
Chekiang Branch
Chinese Medical Association

Yü Shih-chün 于诗俊
Secretary General
Chekiang Branch
Chinese Medical Association

Wu Chih-ch'ing 吴芝青
Doctor
Hospital of Traditional Medicine

Wang Chüan-chiang 王全将
Doctor
Hospital of Traditional Medicine

Chu Min-kuei 诸敏奎
Doctor
Chekiang Provincial Institute
of Materia Medica

Yang Hsüeh-yuan 楊学远
Doctor
Chekiang Medical College

Kwangchow

Hu Ko-ming 胡克明
Leading Member
Kwangtung Branch
Chinese Medical Association

Li Ch'un-yu 李春友
Deputy Secretary General
Kwangtung Branch
Chinese Medical Association

Li Jui-fan (Mme) 李瑞範
Deputy Secretary General
Kwangtung Branch
Chinese Medical Association

Teng Hsi-ku 邓锡谷
Professor, Biochemistry Dept.
Chung Shan Medical College

Wu Hsiu-jung (Mme) 吴秀荣
Professor of Pharmacology
Chung Shan Medical College

Liang Sung-ming 梁颂明
Chairman, Pharmacology Dept.
Kwangtung Traditional Medical College

Li Kuo-yuan 李国沅
Staff Member
Kwangtung Branch
Chinese Medical Association

Chung Chih-ch'ang 鍾智昌
Interpreter
Kwangtung Branch
Chinese Medical Association

Huang Pai-hsin 黄百欣
Interpreter
Kwangtung Branch
China International Travel Service

Persons attending a welcoming banquet in Peking

Yen Chün 阎钧
Leading Member
Chinese Medical Association

Hu Cheng-k'ai 胡正凱
Vice Chairman
Revolutionary Committee
Institute of Materia Medica

Fu Feng-yung 傅丰永
Head of Dept. of Phytochemistry
Institute of Materia Medica

Han Jui 韓锐
Head of Dept. of Pharmacology
Institute of Materia Medica

Sung Chen-yü 宋振玉
Professor of Pharmacology
Institute of Materia Medica

Yang Kuang 杨光
Leading Member
Peking Medical Association

Chang K'uei 张奎
Leading Member
Institute of Chinese Materia Medica

Chao Jung-lai 赵荣莱
Chief of Internal Medicine
Peking Hospital of Chinese
Traditional Medicine

K'ou Wen-jung 寇文镕
Doctor of Internal Medicine
Fu Wai Hospital

Yu Tsu-yuan 余祖元
Staff Member
Foreign Ministry

(In addition, the following people attended a banquet given in return by the group)

Wu Ying-k'ai 吴英恺
Director
Fu Wai Hospital

Wu Huan-hsing 吴桓兴
Director
Jih T'an Hospital

Lo Hui-yuan 罗会元
Doctor of Internal Medicine
Jih T'an Hospital

George Hatem (Ma Hai-teh)
American doctor resident of Peking
Dermatologist at Fu Wai Hospital

Appendix E

Institutions Visited - Brief Descriptions

Kuang An Men Hospital, Peking 广安门医院

Director	Shih Hsiu-chang	師绣章
Surgeon	Li Chih-chung	李志中
Obstetrician	Chang Ta-jung	張大荣
Opthamologist	T'an Yu-chih	唐由之
Urologist	Chia Chin-ming	贾金銘

This is the most important of the three hospitals which are affiliated with the Institute of Chinese Materia Medica, which is part of the Academy of Traditional Chinese Medicine. Established 19 years ago as an outpatient hospital, it now has 160 beds and serves 2000 outpatients per day. There are 116 doctors, 35 of whom are Chinese traditional doctors and 81 of whom are Western-trained doctors who have studied Chinese medicine. Hospital departments include acupuncture, opthamology, urology, surgery, orthopedics, internal medicine, and dermatology.

Institute of Chinese Materia Medica Academy of Chinese Traditional Medicine, Peking 中医研究院中药研究所

Leading Member	Chang K'uei	张奎
Leading Member	Chang Kuo-chen	章国镇
Leading Member, 1st Research Dept.	Hsieh Tsung-wan	谢宗万
Leading Member, 2nd Research Dept.	Yü Kuo-yuan	余国媛
Leading Member 3rd Research Dept.	Ching Hou-te	景厚德
Leading Member 4th Research Dept.	Liu Ching-ming	刘静明

The four research sections, whose leading members are identified above, are: 1) identification and processing of herbs, 2) development of dosage forms, 3) chemical research on traditional drugs, and 4) pharmacological research on traditional drugs. The institute was established in 1955 and has a staff of 150, of whom 130 are scientific and technical personnel.

Peking Hospital of Chinese Traditional Medicine 北京中医医院

Vice Director	Chang Hsiu-lan	张秀兰
Vice Director	Liu Tseng	刘增
Chief, Internal Medicine	Chao Jung-lai	赵荣莱
Deputy Chief, Dept. of Acupuncture and Moxibustion	Ho P'u-jen	贺普仁

This municipal hospital was established in 1956 for the prevention and treatment of disease, teaching, and scientific research. It has a staff of 700 people, of whom 100 are doctors of Chinese traditional medicine and 150 are Western-trained doctors who have studied traditional medicine. The hospital contains 160 beds, but a new facility is being built with room for 240 more beds. It serves 4000-5000 outpatients per day. The departments include internal medicine, surgery, obstetrics and gynecology, pediatrics, and acupuncture. The hospital conducts a medical school which offers a one and a half year course in Chinese traditional medicine for Western-trained doctors.

Fu Wai Hospital, Peking 阜外医院

Director; Professor of Cardiovasculascular Diseases and Surgery	Wu Ying-k'ai	吴英恺
Vice Director; Professor of Internal Medicine	Ts'ai Ju-sheng	蔡如升
Deputy Chief, Internal Medicine	Liu Li-sheng	刘力生
Attending Doctor of Internal Medicine	K'ou Wen-jung	寇文镕
Head Nurse	Yang Ying-hua	杨英华
Chief, Dept. of Pharmacology	Ch'ou Chen-han	仇振涵

This hospital was established in 1958 and now has 350 beds. It is a general hospital of medium or small size for those who live in the area, but the stress is on cardiovascular disease, to which 60-70% of the effort is devoted. In clinical research the areas are: heart disease, hypertension, chronic bronchitis, and pulmonary disease.

Peking University 北京大学
Department of Organic Chemistry and Biochemistry

Organic Chemist	Chang Fan	张凡
Organic Chemist	Chang Ming-che	张明哲
Biochemist	Lin Chien	林建
Biochemist	Shen T'ung	沈同

The University itself was established in 1898 and has been a leading center of learning. After the Cultural Revolution it has undergone changes in curriculum and orientation. At present there are 20 faculties with 75 specialties including social sciences, natural sciences, and foreign languages. Students are accepted upon recommendation by their fellow workers, peasants, or soldiers after having spent at least two years in practical experince after graduation from junior middle school. The length of study has been reduced from four-five years to three years except in some specialties such as theoretical physics or Arabic languages, where it is four years. Teaching methods now reflect the trend toward combining theory with practice. The faculty of natural sciences has established seven factories and has working relationships with 65 factories outside the university.

The first group of 2300 students was graduated in January 1974, having entered the university in January 1971. About 150 have remained to become teacher-candidates. Since 1970 the university has accepted 5600 students in regular programs and 7000 students in short-term courses.

Institute of Materia Medica 中国医学科学院药物研究所
Chinese Academy of Medical Sciences, Peking

Vice Chairman, Revolutionary Committee	Hu Cheng-k'ai	胡正凯
Professor of Pharmacology	Sung Chen-yü	宋振玉
Professor, Synthetic Chemistry Dept.	Liang Hsiao-t'ien	梁晓天
Leading Member, Dept. of Phytochemistry	Fu Feng-yung	傅丰永
Leading Member, Dept of Medicinal Plants	Hsiao P'ei-ken	蕭培根
Leading Member, Dept. of Pharmacology	Han Jui	韓銳
Responsible Person, Office of Scientific Research	Chang Chün-t'ien	张均田

The institute was established in 1958 and has a staff of 300 scientific and technical personnel. Its objectives are to seek new drugs to prevent and treat the most common diseases and to do research on drugs and drug principles which have been proved to be effective practically. The four areas of emphasis are: treatment of the common cold and bronchitis, treatment of tumors, treatment of cardiovascular disease, and contraception.

The institute is organized into seven departments: Synthetic drugs, Phytochemistry, Pharmacology, Chemical analysis of drugs, Medicinal plants, Antibiotics, and Cultivation of medicinal plants. An experimental plantation in the Peking suburbs is under the direction of the cultivation of medicinal plants department.

Experimental Plantation
Institute of Materia Medica, Peking

This botanical garden, which encompasses an area of about 400 Mou and includes about 1500 species under cultivation, is under the direction of the cultivation and medicinal plants department of the Institute of Materia Medica in Peking. The garden itself is located on the outskirts of the city. The leading member of the facility is Hsiao P'ei-ken, a pharmacognosist. The functions of the plantation are:

1. to introduce the cultivation of herbs from China and abroad.

2. to improve cultivation by decreasing growing time and by the prevention and treatment of plant disease and insects.

3. to cultivate seedlings.

4. to gather information on Chinese medicinal herbs and to make positive identification of each species when the plants were known previously only under the vernacular name.

5. to supply research laboratories with sufficient authenticated plant material for biological evaluations or phytochemical studies.

6. to maintain adequate seed supplies (germ plasm) of as many medicinal plants as possible.

7. to train barefoot doctors in identifying the most important medicinal plants.

Jih T'an Hospital, Peking 日壇医院

Director,	Wu Huan-hsing	吴桓兴
Vice Director Revolutionary Committee	Li Ping	李冰
Doctor of Internal Medicine	Lo Hui-yuan	罗会元
Chief, Radiology Department	Ku Hsien-chih	谷铣之
Doctor of Internal Medicine	Sun Yen	孫燕
Leading member, Office of Scientific Research	Cheng Ya-ming	郑亚明

This hospital is also the tumor prevention research institute of the Chinese Academy of Medical Sciences. It is responsible for coordinating the research work throughout China on esophageal cancer.

Nan-K'ai Hospital, Tientsin 南开医院

Vice Director	Wu Hsien-chung	吴咸中
Chief, Internal Medicine	Chao Ssu-chien	赵思儉
Deputy Chief, Surgery Dept.	Lo Lien-cheng	罗连成

This is a general hospital for the Nan-K'ai district of Tientsin, built in 1952, and now contains 320 beds. The staff numbers 418 doctors, nurses, and technicians, and treats 1500 outpatients per day. A principal area of research is the non-operative treatment of acute abdominal diseases. Doctors at Nan-K'ai are able to treat about 70% of their patients with acute abdominal diseases through a combination of Western and Chinese traditional medicine without using surgery. For example, about 80% of the cases of acute appendicitis and 70% of the cases of perforated acute ulcer are treated non-surgically in this manner. The hospital also trains those doctors who have received a Western-oriented medical education in Chinese traditional medicine.

Tientsin Hospital, Tientsin 天津医院

Director	Ma T'u-wei 馬突围
Chief, Dept. of Orthopedics	T'ao Fu 陶甫
Deputy Chief, Dept. of Orthopedics	Shang T'ien-yü 尚天裕

This hospital has five clinical departments: internal medicine, surgery, gynecology, Chinese traditional medicine, and orthopedics. There are 600 beds, of which 350 are devoted to orthopedics. About 1500 outpatients are treated each day. Since 1958 the hospital has specialized in a new treatment of bone fractures. After administering acupuncture analgesia, doctors reduce the fracture by manipulation. Then they immobilize the fractured bone with splints, leaving the joints on both ends free, and prescribe exercises for the patient. This mobility apparently facilitates the union of the bone and shortens the course of treatment by 50%. It also is said to prevent complications often seen with other methods.

Capital Hospital, Peking 首都医院

Chief, Surgery Dept.	Feng Ch'uan-I 馮传宜
Deputy Chief, Internal Medicine	Chin Lan 金兰
Deputy Chief Gynecology Dept.	Lien Li-chüan 连利娟
Professor of Gynecology	Sung Hung-chao 宋鸿钊
Responsible Person, Administrative Dept.	Lo Ling 羅铃

Formerly known as the Peking Union Medical College, the Capital Hospital is located about two blocks off a main shopping street, Wang Fu Ching. It is a general hospital, with 550 beds, and is the center for treatment of foreign residents and guests in Peking. The three principal departments are internal medicine, surgery, and gynecology. There are about 60 physicians in postgraduate training in the hospital each year. There is also a nursing school with 60 students.

The Library of the Chinese Academy of Medical Sciences is located within the hospital. It has a collection of over 300,000 volumes, and has subscriptions to 1400 journals, including foreign journals.

Shanghai Institute of Materia Medica 上海药物研究所

Leading Member, Revolutionary Committee	Tuan Hsün-fu	段勳復
Chief, Dept. of Synthetic Chemistry	Kao I-sheng	高怡生
Deputy Chief, Dept. of Synthetic Chemistry	Chi Ju-ch'en	嵇汝臣
Chief, Phytochemistry Dept.	Hsu Jen-sheng	徐任生
Chief, Pharmacology Dept.	Hsu Pin	胥彬

Originally part of the Chinese Academy of Sciences, this institute is now under the direction of the Municipal Revolutionary Committee of Shanghai. There are 470 staff members, of whom 300 are research personnel. The five departments are: Synthetic drugs, Phytochemistry, Pharmacology, Analytical chemistry, and Antibiotics.

The main tasks of the institute are to study new drugs in the areas of cancer, nervous diseases, liver diseases, cardiovascular diseases, chronic bronchitis, hepatitis, and contraception. The approaches involve synthetic drugs and materials isolated from plants and microorganisms. For known drugs from the West, the work is directed to better routes for synthesis and to modification of extraction procedures appropriate for isolation of compounds from Chinese plants. Little pure biochemical or physiological research is done in the institute, although some basic work is being undertaken in support of the applied projects in drug synthesis or drug metabolism.

Lung Hua Hospital of Traditional Medicine, Shanghai

Established in 1960, this is a general hospital of Chinese Traditional medicine, with 250 beds and 2000 outpatients per day. The staff numbers 400, of whom 100 are physicians and 100 are nurses. Every year about 40-50 medical personnel are sent to the countryside and factories to treat the common diseases, train barefoot doctors and worker doctors, and to receive re-education.

Shanghai #2 Pharmaceutical Factory of Traditional Chinese Drugs

This factory produces over 30 products using herbs as raw materials. Established in 1958 with a staff of only 80, it now has a work force of 470 and prepares tablets, pills, liquids, and granules made from extracts.

The following processes were viewed by the Herbal Pharmacology Study Group:

1. preparation of liquid extract

2. coating of pills with fluid extract and solid extract

3. preparation of granules by mixing a concentrated alcoholic extract of crude drug with sugar and drying after passing through a coarse sieve. This is dissolved in hot water by the patient who drinks it as a tea for asthma.

4. tableting of powdered extract on high speed rotary presses. Apparently the standard formula includes starch as disintegrant or binder and talc as lubricant.

5. sugar coating of tablets in large pans about the same size used in the U.S.

6. packaging

Nanking College of Pharmacy, Nanking

This is a relatively small school, established in 1936 with 42 students and a faculty of six full-time and five part-time. Through 1948 they averaged 30 graduates per year and the curriculum required four years. From 1949-1952 it was known as the East China School of Pharmacy, but it enrolled students from all over the country. Prior to the Cultural Revolution, the curriculum was five years with two specialty areas: chemistry and pharmacy.

Since the Cultural Revolution, there have been many changes. During 1972 and 1973 the college enrolled a total of 530 students in two specialty areas: pharmacy and pharmaceutical chemistry. The curriculum was shortened from five years to three years; the courses have been both reduced and simplified. Students are admitted from among the workers, peasants, and soldiers who have practical experience following graduation from middle school. The system of education was described as "open door education," in which close contacts are maintained between the school and the factories in order to combine theory with practice and to prevent education from being divorced from reality. Students spend a period annually in the factories, hospitals, or in the countryside.

Research is closely related to practical need. Graduates of the pharmaceutical chemistry curriculum go to work in factories in chemical synthesis. Pharmacy graduates work in factories and drug control laboratories. Some stay on to become teachers.

In addition to the Nanking College of Pharmacy, there is an independent pharmacy college in Shenyang. There are also three faculties of pharmacy associated with medical colleges in Peking, Shanghai, and Chengtu.

Kiangsu Provincial Hospital of Chinese Traditional Medicine, Nanking 江苏省中医医院

Chairman, Revolutionary Committee	Chang Chih-hua	张治华
Chief, Internal Medicine	Hsu Ch'ang-kuei	徐长桂
Chief, Acupuncture and Moxibustion Dept.	Ch'iu Mao-liang	邱茂良
Chief, Pharmacy Dept.	Sun Hao-nien	孫鶴年
Traditional Doctor	Chiang Lin-yu	蒋淋右
Traditional Pharmacist	Chiang Chin-hsiang	姜金祥

This hospital was established in 1954 and now has 300 beds. About 2000 outpatients are treated per day. There are nine departments: internal medicine, surgery, gynecology, pediatrics, acupuncture, opthamology, proctology, massage, and dermatology. In most cases, Chinese traditional medicine and drugs are used in treatment, but Western drugs are also used. It was said that sometimes Western drugs are used in emergency and Chinese traditional drugs are used for consolidation. There is also some emphasis on use of newer dosage forms of Chinese traditional drugs, instead of decoction, for the convenience of the patient.

Jui Chin Hospital, Shanghai 瑞金医院

Responsible Member, Revolutionary Committee	Shih P'u-chai	时朴斋
Doctor, Dept. of Burn	Hsü Wei-shih	许偉石
Doctor, Dept. of Orthopedics	Ch'ien Pu-fan	钱不凡
Doctor, Dept. of Orthopedics	Ch'ü Ke-fu	曲克服
Chairman, Dept of Acupuncture and Moxibustion	Ch'en Ta-chung	陳大中

This is a teaching hospital of the Shanghai Second Medical College. It has 1100 beds and sees, on the average, 3000 outpatients per day and on some days up to 4000. The staff of 1700 includes 350 physicians, 400 nurses, and 200 technicians working in 19 medical departments, including burn treatment and acupuncture, and nine auxiliary departments (laboratory, x-ray, etc.). In surgery, acupuncture analgesia is used quite extensively, i.e. in about 50% of the cases, with 80% success.

Hua Shan Hospital, Shanghai 上海第一医学院附属华山医院

Responsible Member, Revolutionary Committee; Surgeon	Chu Hsi-ch'i 朱锡琪
Responsible Member, Pharmacy	Ch'en Hsiang-ying 陳湘英
Doctor of Internal Medicine	Tai Jui-hung 戴瑞鸿

This is a teaching hospital of the Shanghai First Medical College. Among its departments is a neurological clinic.

Institute of Organic Chemistry, Chinese Academy of Sciences, Shanghai 上海科学院上海有机化学研究所

Deputy Director	Wang Yu 汪猷
Professor; Responsible Member, Dept. of Natural Organic Chemistry	Liu Chu-chin 刘铸晋
Professor; Responsible Member, Dept of Natural Organic Chemistry	Chou Wei-shan 周维善
Professor; Responsible Member, Dept. of Fluoride Compounds	Huang Wei-yuan 黄維垣

The institute was established in 1950 with a staff of four people. Prior to that time there was no institute specializing in organic chemistry. At the beginning research was closely related to rehabilitation of the country, e.g. in antibiotics, polymers, and herbal drugs. In 1958 the latter group was split off and became the Institute of Materia Medica in Shanghai. Now there are 1100 workers in the four main areas of the institute: Chemistry of natural organic products, Elementary organic chemistry, Chemistry of extractives, and Biological, analytical, and physical chemistry.

Current work of the institute includes total synthesis of insulin, synthesis of nucleic acids, petroleum microbial oxidation, steroid hormones and oral contraceptives, and organic fluorine chemistry.

About one-third of the institute's technical staff is concerned with various aspects of natural products chemistry. Of these, 30 chemists have been assigned to nucleotide chemistry, 17 to polypeptide chemistry and others seemed concerned with steroid development (oral contraceptives), synthesis of protein sources, and fluorine polymer chemistry (for example, polytetrafluoroethylene).

Kwangtung Botanical Garden, Kwangchow 廣東植物园

Leading Member, Revolutionary Committee	Ts'ui Kuo-cheng	崔国成
Leading Member, Forestry Dept.	Kuan Hsüeh-liang	关学良
Leading Member, Forestry Dept.	Shao Ying-shao	邵应韶
Leading Member, Seed Development Dept.	Chu Chan-ch'ang	朱湛昌
Staff Member, Administrative Office	Yeh Yü-yen	葉玉燕

The purposes of this facility are to indroduce, cultivate, propagate, and produce plants for research and teaching purposes. The area of the garden was approximately 3000 Mou, with about 3000 species under cultivation. The facility employs 120 workers.

Kwangtung College of Chinese Traditional Medicine, Kwangchow 廣東中医学院

Vice Chairman, Revolutionary Committee	Li Fu-hai	李福海
Vice Chairman, Educational Revolution Group and Chairman Dept. of Internal Medicine	Teng T'ieh-t'ao	邓铁涛
Vice Chairman, Educational Revolution Group	Ou Ming	欧明
Deputy Chairman, Dept. of Trauma	Huang Yao-hsin	黄耀燊
Deputy Chairman, Dept. of Trauma	Mai Kuan-min	麦冠民
Deputy Chairman, Dept. of Acupuncture & Moxibustion	Chin Jui	靳瑞

Deputy Chairman, Pharmacy Dept.	Li Hsiu-t'ing	李秀挺
Deputy Chairman, Pharmacy Dept.	Li Jui	李锐
Professor, Pharmacy Dept.	Kao Han-sen	高汉森
Professor, Pharmacy Dept.	Wu Ch'iao-I	吴俏仪
Chief, Office of Scientific Research	Chang Shu-min	张淑敏

Since its establishment in 1956 until the beginning of the Cultural Revolution in 1966, the college enrolled 1100 students and 130 doctors trained in Western medicine. Since the Cultural Revolution, the school enrolls 200-300 students per year and 200 Western-trained doctors. Among the students are barefoot doctors. Disciplines have been reduced from 36 to 14, and the curriculum from 6 to 3 years. About 25% of the students are women. Graduates, who are called "doctors of traditional Chinese medicine," go mainly to factories and communes; some go to hospitals. In the new curriculum, about 210 hours is devoted to traditional drugs and about 60 hours to Western drugs.

Chung Shan Medical College, Kwangchow

Vice Chairman Revolutionary Committee	Yao Ts'ung-jen	姚崇仁
Associate Professor of Biochemistry	Hsü Hsiao-li	徐晓利
Associate Professor of Pharmacology	Wu Hsiu-jung	吴秀荣
Doctor of Traditional Medicine	Hsieh T'ing-ch'i	谢庭启
Leading Member, Educational Revolution Committee	Ho Tzu-ch'ien	何子谦
Instructor, Phytochemistry Dept.	Wang Mei-ching	王玫静
Member, Revolutionary Committee	Huang Huan-hsin	黄焕新

Vice Chairman, Revolutionary Committee First Affiliated Hosp.	Wu Han-pang	伍汉邦
Vice Chairman, Revolutionary Committee, Tumor Hospital	Tu Kuan-I	杜冠一
Chairman, Head & Neck Dept., Tumor Hospital	Li Chen-ch'üan	李振权
Attending Doctor, First Affiliated Hospital	Mai Kuo-chien	麦国建
Traditional Doctor, First Affiliated Hospital	Ch'iu Jui-hsiang	丘瑞香

Chung Shan Medical College was established in 1953 on the basis of three older medical schools: the faculty of medicine of Lingnan University, the faculty of medicine of Chung Shan University, and the Kuang Hua Medical College. There are five hospitals affiliated with the College, three of which are general hospitals, one a tumor hospital, and one an eye hospital. They total 2100 beds.

There are now 1200 students in the first two years of the post-Cultural Revolution curriculum and 600 more will be admitted in the fall of 1974. The faculty numbers 800, of whom 30 are in pharmacology. There is also a two-year nursing school with an enrollment of 120.

Following the practice of dispensing with entrance exams, the school admits workers, peasants, and soldiers who have had practical experience following graduation from junior middle school. Students must be unmarried and in good health, and have demonstrated a good knowledge of Marxism-Leninism.

The College adheres to the policy of Mao Tse-tung of "open-door education" which stresses the following:

1. maintain contact between the college and the commune and county hospitals; send students and faculty there to provide medical care and to learn to serve the people.

2. establish a teaching base in the countryside, with classrooms and laboratories; send mobile medical teams there to provide care, train barefoot doctors.

3. reduce the curriculum by: a) reducing the length of study from six years to three years to meet the needs of the people to train as many doctors as possible; b) simplify the courses from 36 down to 15 by removing duplicates and unnecessary subjects; c) changing the method of teaching by integrating theory with practice, preclinical with clinical, Chinese with Western medicine, treatment with prevention.

Upon entering the college, the student spends six months in review courses, which include politics, foreign languages, math, physics, chemistry, etc. That is, the student enters the review course in April. In October, the first year of medical school begins, with the following curriculum:

Year I: Function and structure of Human Body
Anatomy, histology, biochemistry, physiology, parasitology, microbiology, pathology, pharmacology

Year II: Diagnosis, internal medicine, surgery, ob-gyn pediatrics, ENT, dermatology, traditional medicine
Students and faculty spend time in the countryside learning public health and hygiene

Year III: Study of medicine through contact with patients; every student looks after 5-10 patients
Pre-clinical courses
Recent advances in medicine
Clinical pathology and clinical pharmacology

The curriculum in pharmacology includes 84 hours (56 lecture, 28 lab) at the end of the first year and 20 hours of clinical pharmacology in the third year.

LIST OF REFERENCES

INTRODUCTION

Page 2 [1]Cooper, William C., and Nathan Sivin. "Man as a medicine: pharmacological and ritual aspects of traditional therapy using drugs derived from the human body." In Shigeru Nakayama and Nathan Sivin, Chinese science: exploration of an ancient tradition. Cambridge, MIT Press, 1073, p. 206.

[2]Croizier, Ralph C. Traditional medicine in modern China: science, nationalism, and the tensions of cultural change. Cambridge, Harvard University Press, 1968. p. 156.

Page 3 [3]Ibid., p. 184.

[4]Cooper and Sivin, op. cit., p. 270.

Page 4 [5]Ibid., p. 203.

[6]Mao Tse-tung. Selected Works. New York, International Publishers, 1954. Vol. I, p. 290.

Page 5 [7]An editorial in the Lancet for May 25, 1975 ("Cancer in Chinese Migrants." p. 1027) summarizes the rather stricking differences between Chinese and non-Chinese in regard to cancers of various sorts, some of which differences disappear when Chinese migrate from their homeland.

Page 6 [8]Hyman, P. and Westring, D.W. Leukocytosis in Acute Appendicitis. JAMA, 229: p. 1630-1631, 1974.

[9]Bonica, J.J. Therapeutic Acupuncture in the People's Republic of China. JAMA, 228: p. 1455-1554, 1974.

Page 7 [10]McCurdy, P.R. B_{12} Shots. JAMA, 229: p. 703-704, 1974.

THE CLINICAL USE OF HERBAL MEDICINES

Page 13 [1]Acute Abdominal Conditions Research Group, Nan K'ai Hospital, Tientsin. "Some problems in nonoperative treatment of acute appendicitis; analysis of immediate and long-term results in 995 cases." Chinese Medical Journal, no. 2, Feb. 1974: p. 21.

Page 15 [2]Nan K'ai Hospital, Tientsin. "Traditional-Western combined treatment of acute perforation of peptic ulcer." Chinese Medical Journal, no. 2, Feb. 1974: p. 20.

Page 25 [3]Bonica, John J. "Therapeutic acupuncture in the People's Republic of China: implications for American medicine." JAMA, Vol. 228, June 17, 1974: p. 1544.

[4]Hsu, R.C. "The Barefoot Doctors of the People's Republic of China--Some Problems." New England Journal of Medicine, 291: p. 124-127, 1974.

Page 26 [5]Cherkasky, Martin. "Health Care Organization and Health Policy Issues." Report of the Medical Delegation to the People's Republic of China. Sponsored by the Committee on Scholarly Communication with the People's Republic of China, June 15 - July 16, 1973. Washington, D.C., National Academy of Sciences, Institute of Medicine. p. 30.

DRUG CONTROL IN CHINA

Page 66 [1]Oksenberg, Michel. "Methods of communication within the Chinese bureaucracy." China quarterly, no. 57, Jan./Mar. 1974: p. 1-39.

[2]Winckler, Edwin. "Political management of the development process: assessing the Chinese development experience." China quarterly, no. 55, July/Sept. 1973: p. 564.